Pediatric High-Alert Medications

Evidence-Based Safe Practices for Nursing Professionals

Jill Duncan, RN, MS, MPH
Jason Corcoran, PharmD, BCPS

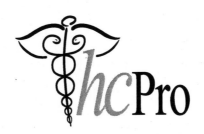

Jill Duncan, RN, MS, MPH, Author

Jason Corcoran, PharmD, BCPS, Author

Rebecca Hendren, Senior Managing Editor

Jamie Gisonde, Executive Editor

Emily Sheahan, Group Publisher

Laura Godinho, Cover Designer

Jackie Diehl Singer, Graphic Artist

Audrey Doyle, Copyeditor

Lauren Rubenzahl, Proofreader

Jean St. Pierre, Director of Operations

Susan Darbyshire, Art Director

Claire Cloutier, Production Manager

Darren Kelly, Books Production Supervisor

Paul Singer, Layout Artist

Advice given is general. Readers should consult professional counsel for specific legal, ethical, or clinical questions.

Arrangements can be made for quantity discounts. For more information, contact:

HCPro, Inc.
P.O. Box 1168
Marblehead, MA 01945
Telephone: 800/650-6787 or 781/639-1872
Fax: 781/639-2982
E-mail: *customerservice@hcpro.com*

Visit HCPro at its World Wide Web sites:

www.hcpro.com and *www.hcmarketplace.com*

21310
11/2007

Contents

About the authors vi

Introduction viii

Chapter 1: What makes pediatric patients different? 1

Introduction 1

Differences in pediatric patients 2

Differences in providing medications to pediatric patients... 5

Differences in medication safety.. 10

Chapter 2: General pediatric medication safety principles 11

What are high-alert medications?.. 11

National Patient Safety Goals 16

Identifying and reporting errors is critical to safety improvement................................... 24

Chapter 3: Technology that improves safety practices 27

New technology 27

Chapter 4: Safely preparing, dispensing, and administering medication to kids of all ages 33

Safe preparation and dispensing.. 33

Safe administration 34

Keep kids safe 44

Chapter 5: Anticoagulation medications 47

Why are anticoagulant medications identified as pediatric high-alert medications?.......... 47

Therapeutic options 48

Who is at risk?.. 49

Pediatric considerations 49

Unfractionated heparin 52

Nursing implications 52

Low molecular weight heparins 55

Nursing implications... 55

Warfarin 58

Nursing implications 59

Miscellaneous anticoagulation therapies 61

Chapter 6: Chemotherapy agents **63**

Why are chemotherapeutic agents identified as pediatric high-alert medications? 63

Therapeutic options 64

Who is at risk? 64

Pediatric considerations 68

Drug-specific information 71

Nursing implications 72

Chapter 7: Concentrated electrolytes **77**

Why are concentrated electrolytes identified as pediatric high-alert medications? 77

Therapeutic options 78

Who is at risk? 81

Pediatric considerations 82

Drug-specific information 84

Nursing implications 87

Chapter 8: Cardiovascular medications **91**

Why are some cardiovascular medications identified as pediatric high-alert medications? 91

Therapeutic options 92

Who is at risk? 92

Pediatric considerations 94

Drug-specific information 96

Nursing implications 98

Patient and family education highlights 101

Chapter 9: Insulin and concentrated dextrose solutions **103**

Why are insulin and concentrated dextrose solutions identified as

pediatric high-alert medications? 103

Therapeutic options with concentrated dextrose solutions 104

Who is at risk with concentrated dextrose solutions? 106

Pediatric considerations with concentrated dextrose solutions 107

Drug-specific information 108

Nursing implications with concentrated dextrose solution 109

Patient and family education highlights 110

Therapeutic options with insulin 111

Who is at risk with insulin? 112

Pediatric considerations with insulin 113

Drug-specific information with insulin 114

Nursing implications with insulin 115

Patient and family education highlights with insulin 116

Chapter 10: Neuromuscular blocking agents **117**

Why are NMBs identified as pediatric high-alert medications? 117

Therapeutic options 119

Who is at risk? 119

Pediatric considerations 120

Drug-specific information 122

Nursing implications 123

Patient and family education highlights 125

Chapter 11: Pediatric pain and sedation medications **127**

Why are some pediatric pain and sedation agents

identified as high-alert medications? 127

Therapeutic options 128

Who is at risk? 129

Pediatric considerations 130

Drug-specific information 132

Nursing implications 134

Pain management safety considerations 135

General pediatric sedation principles 137

Sedation safety considerations 139

Bibliography **143**

Nursing education instructional guide **151**

Continuing education exam 157

Continuing education evaluation 167

About the authors

Jill Duncan, RN, MS, MPH

Jill Duncan, RN, MS, MPH, is the clinical nurse specialist for the neonatal intensive care unit (NICU) at Inova Fairfax Hospital for Children in Falls Church, VA. She has more than 14 years of pediatric-related experience in a variety of acute care settings, including the National Institutes of Health (NIH).

Duncan began her career working with adult and pediatric neurology and neurosurgery patients at NIH. After gaining valuable experience in the inpatient research setting, she transitioned to work with acutely ill neonates and their families in a host of large tertiary care medical centers. She eventually expanded her NICU experience to include work in a Level I trauma pediatric emergency department, as well as pediatric and neonatal transport. In her current role, she supports the NICU's participation in the Vermont Oxford Network's Evidence-Based Quality Improvement Collaborative and plays a significant leadership role in her unit's work related to clinical practice improvement and patient safety initiatives.

She received her master's of science and master's of public health degrees with a focus in maternal and child health from the University of Illinois at Chicago in 2000 and her bachelor of science in nursing from Georgetown University in Washington, DC, in 1993. Her professional memberships include the National Association of Neonatal Nurses and The Academy of Neonatal Nursing. She was featured in an Academy of Neonatal Nursing member spotlight in 2007. The same publication also highlighted the collaborative work she has done on the development of a virtual NICU critical decision simulation education program for nurses. She is also an active volunteer with the March of Dimes, National Capital Area Chapter.

Jason Corcoran, PharmD, BCPS

Jason Corcoran, PharmD, BCPS, is the clinical pharmacy specialist for the Inova Fairfax Hospital for Children in Falls Church, VA. He has more than 10 years of pharmacy work experience, including the past five years in practice as a pediatric pharmacist.

Corcoran began his career as a pharmacy technician in his hometown of Richmond, VA, and an interest in the unique aspects of providing medications to children led him to pursue post-graduate residency training.

After completing hospital pharmacy practice and pediatric specialty residencies at The Johns Hopkins Hospital based in Baltimore in 2003, he was a clinical pharmacy specialist in the pediatric intensive care unit at the Children's Hospital, Cleveland OH Clinic. While at the Cleveland Clinic, Corcoran took part in many safety initiatives, most notably in the implementation of standardized continuous infusions.

In his current role at Inova Fairfax, he provides clinical pharmacy oversight for 186 pediatric beds comprising the pediatric intensive care, neonatal intensive care, pediatric medical-surgical, pediatric hematology-oncology, pediatric emergency, and adolescent units. This role allows him to see the unique medication safety needs across all pediatric subspecialties. His participation in several hospital and systemwide safety teams has also allowed him to play a key role in the implementation of important safety initiatives such as standardized continuous infusions, smart-pump technology, and prior approval of off-label, high-risk medication use in pediatrics.

Corcoran received his doctor of pharmacy degree from Virginia Commonwealth University based in Richmond in 2001. He is a member of pharmaceutical organizations including the American Society of Health Systems Pharmacists and the American College of Clinical Pharmacy. As a member of the Pediatric Pharmacy Advocacy Group for the past five years, he has twice been invited to speak at its national meetings. In 2005 he achieved board-certification in pharmacotherapy, a qualification that recognizes additional knowledge, experience, and skills in a defined area of pharmacy practice.

Introduction

Concern surrounding pediatric high-alert medications has garnered increased attention from institutions and organizations nationwide. Professional associations, regulatory bodies, and even the news media have all targeted safety, especially medication safety, as a significant problem in today's healthcare system. This increased attention stems from mounting awareness surrounding the unique needs of pediatric patients, together with a growing body of literature that demonstrates an increased number of errors occurring in the pediatric population (AAP Policy Statement 2003; Alton et al. 2006; Hughes and Edgerton 2005; Levine et al. 2001). Studies also suggest increased morbidity following medication errors or adverse events in pediatric patients compared to adults (AAP Policy Statement 2003; Alton et al. 2006; Hughes and Edgerton 2005; Levine et al. 2001).

Safe dosing, dispensing, and administration of pediatric high-alert medications requires a multidisciplinary, multisystem approach to medication safety. Although most documented errors, such as dosing errors or transcription mistakes, occur before a medication is administered to the patient, nurses play a significant role in pediatric medication safety (Fortescue, et al. 2003). Nurses are the ones who most frequently administer medications to patients; they are often the last layer of protection or potential barrier between a medication error and the potential for serious harm to the patient (Hughes and Edgerton 2005).

Our hope is that this book will improve pediatric high-alert medication safety. Information addressed includes national patient safety initiatives and alerts, evidence-based research, some basic pharmacology principles, and practical clinical experience aimed at raising awareness of not only high-alert safety practices, but also of how high-alert medication safety practices can be integrated into pediatric nursing care.

The introductory chapters aim to describe the unique features of pediatric patients, as well as to provide a review of national safety initiatives and emerging safety technologies and an introduction to medication safety principles unique to pediatric patients and their families. The chapters that follow address seven different pediatric high-alert medication classes. Each high-alert medication chapter includes an overview of the basic pharmacology principles, administration and safety concerns specific to pediatric patients, and examples of errors and good catches surrounding high-alert medication practices.

Empowering patients and their families by teaching them about the ways they can play a part in medication safety is often an overlooked resource in our quest to improve safe processes. Therefore, we also aim to impress upon the reader the importance of involving children and their families in their own safety, in ways that fit their stage of development and current healthcare needs.

The case studies included often demonstrate devastating and even fatal errors. The intention is not to focus solely on what went wrong, or who was at fault, but rather for readers to learn from the mistakes and begin to think about how to prevent similar errors from occurring in their own practices. It is also not our intention for the information included in this book to serve as a clinical resource for daily dosing and administration. Although we address some medication-specific information, our intent is to support the safety principles described rather than to serve as an approved pharmacology handbook. In fact, we purposefully left out specific pediatric dosing, compatibility, and administration guidelines to reinforce the necessity of using approved references as clinical resources, especially when it comes to pediatric high-alert medications.

As healthcare professionals charged with caring for children of all ages, we are deeply committed to improving the safety of the care we provide. Many of the devastating, and even fatal, outcomes stemming from pediatric high-alert medication errors could have been prevented. We hope this overview of current standards, trends, and clinical information affecting pediatric high-alert medication safety will drive those who care for children to become passionate about keeping these children—and their families—safe.

—Jill Duncan, RN, MS, MPH, and Jason Corcoran, PharmD, BCPS

Chapter 1 | What makes pediatric patients different?

Learning objectives

After reading this chapter, the reader will be able to:

- Identify the key differences in providing pharmaceutical care to pediatric patients

- Recognize the importance of a systems approach to medication safety in pediatric patients

- Explain the special considerations necessary when formulating adult dosage forms for pediatric administration

Introduction

It is no secret that medication use in pediatric patients is different than with adults. What can seem like a secret is how to best care for this different population. Most formalized education is centered on caring for adult patients, and many efforts to protect patients from medication errors do not include pediatric-specific considerations. But the uniqueness of pediatric patients can increase the likelihood and seriousness of medication errors (Lesar 1998; Kaushal 2001).

The pediatric patient population is diverse and can include everyone from a 0.4 kg baby to a 110 kg obese teenager. To better care for such a diverse population, it helps to be able to classify

| Figure 1.1 | What makes pediatric patients different? |

Group	Age
Premature neonate	<38 weeks gestational age at birth
Neonate (newborn)	Birth to one month
Infant (baby)	One month to one year
Young child	One to five years
Older child	Six to 12 years
Adolescent	Thirteen to 18 years

"pediatric" patients based on several age groups. Different references and practitioners may have slightly different age cut-offs, but Figure 1.1 illustrates the most common classifications.

Differences in pediatric patients

Nurses must be cognizant of the many differences between adult and pediatric patients when caring for children.

Size differences

Aside from the obvious difference in weight between children and adults, there are some less obvious size differences. Pediatric patients have increased body mass and body surface area (BSA) per kilogram (kg) than adults (Yaffe 2005). In addition, organs such as the brain, liver, and kidneys are proportionally larger in pediatric patients (Yaffe 2005). Although larger children may approach adult weight, the other size differences may not disappear until after adolescents have gone through puberty (Yaffe 2005).

Pharmacokinetic differences

Absorption: Decreased gastric emptying time, immature biliary function, and changes in microflora generally lead to a decrease in absorption compared to adults (Yaffe 2005). However, immature enzymes, increased permeability of the intestine, and increased surface area of the intestine may increase the absorption of some drugs (Yaffe 2005). Gastric pH is generally higher in pediatric patients, but can fluctuate during the early months of development. The effect of gastric pH on drugs is drug-specific, with a higher pH (less acidic) resulting in the increased absorption of acid-labile drugs such as penicillin (Yaffe 2005).

These physiologic differences resolve at different times, and overall gastrointestinal function will mature to adult levels by two years of age (ASHP 2004). Further gastrointestinal complications in adolescents include malabsorption of drugs in patients with anorexic or bulimic disorders or cystic fibrosis. Topical medications may have enhanced absorption in children due to thinner skin and a greater BSA-to-weight ratio. Intramuscular absorption is variable due to decreased muscle mass and increased blood supply to skeletal muscles (ASHP 2004).

Distribution: The percentage of body water in pediatric patients decreases as age increases. Total body water is around 80% of total body weight in newborns, but it decreases to adult levels of 60% midway through the first year of life (Yaffe 2005). This can result in a larger volume of distribution for water-soluble drugs such as aminoglycosides.

There is also an increase in the percentage of body fat in children between the ages of 5 and 10 years (Murphy 2001). This is followed by an increase in lean body mass during adolescence (Murphy 2001). In females, total body water and lean body mass decrease in late puberty, whereas total body water and lean body mass increase throughout puberty in males (Murphy 2001). These changes in body composition can affect both volume of distribution and protein binding. For example, lipid-soluble drugs such as midazolam will have an increased volume of distribution in a 5-year-old with increased percentage of body fat. Plasma protein levels increase to adult levels during childhood. Therefore, some young children may still have increased free fraction of highly protein-bound drugs such as phenytoin.

Metabolism: Phase I (cytochrome P450) enzymes vary greatly with age. Generally, phase I enzymes are immature during infancy, exhibit increased activity during childhood, and then decrease gradually with adult levels being attained at puberty (Yaffe 2005). This increase in enzymatic activity in childhood often requires increases in weight-based dosing. Phase II enzymes also vary in their age-related activity: for acetaminophen metabolism, glucuronidation increases with age, whereas sulfation decreases with age (Murphy 2001). Sometimes, the predominant metabolic pathway of a drug changes with age. For example, the early metabolism of theophylline is accomplished by N_7-methylation rather than oxidative demethylation. As a result, neonates can convert theophylline into caffeine, something coffee-loving adults only wish they could do (Yaffe 2005). Although not well defined, metabolism also can be affected by pharmacogenetics (Yaffe 2005). In other words, a given patient may be genetically predisposed to metabolize certain drugs more slowly or more quickly.

Elimination: Glomerular filtration increases rapidly during the first two weeks of life, with continued improvement to adult values by six to 12 months of age (Murphy 2001). Changes occur later in development as well. Study information with uric acid clearance shows that adults have reduced clearance compared to prepubescent children and adolescents (Yaffe 2005). Another consideration is the effect that certain medications may have on otherwise normal renal function. Nephrotoxic chemotherapy agents such as cyclophosphamide may damage the kidney at therapeutic doses and result in reduced elimination of all renally cleared drugs.

Differences in drug-related problems

Numerous drug-related problems (DRP) are possible in children and adolescents. Children and adolescents are at risk for the same types of DRPs that can affect adults: adverse drug reactions, drug interactions, therapeutic duplications, inappropriate drug selection, subtherapeutic doses, overdoses, untreated indications, no indications, or incorrect administration of medications (ASHP). However, children are at a greater risk for DRPs for a number of reasons:

- Immature organs can result in less protein binding, reduced clearance, and enhanced absorption of medications, all of which can contribute to toxicities in young children

- Small doses that require further dilution, calculations, or partial dosage forms have a greater likelihood of resulting in overdoses or ineffective doses

- There is a lack of standardization and limited information on stability regarding tablets that are compounded into oral suspensions for pediatric patients

- There is a increased risk of toxicity when using dosage forms designed for adults (e.g., transdermal patches)

- Certain toxicities are unique to pediatric patients, such as abnormal development of teeth and bones associated with tetracycline

- Inactive ingredients in medications can pose a problem for pediatric patients:
  - Ethanol (up to 10% in elixirs) can cause intoxication or disulfiram-like reactions
  - Benzyl alcohol can cause metabolic acidosis

- Propylene glycol can cause cardiac arrhythmias or hypotension
- Lactose can cause diarrhea, cramping, bloating, and flatulence in certain patients
- Sucrose can affect blood sugar levels or counteract a ketogenic diet
- Sorbitol can cause diarrhea or cramping if given in large amounts

Children and adolescents have unique barriers to adherence:

- Fear of doctors and medications
- Poor taste of liquid and chewable medications
- Lack of understanding of their disease state and the importance of medication
- Interruptions in dosing schedules due to school and extracurricular activities
- Peer pressure or embarrassment regarding taking medication in front of others

Differences in providing medications to pediatric patients

The differences in pediatric patients require that the provision of medication therapy to children be different as well. It is dangerous when pediatric patients are simply treated as "little adults." For example, a 7-year-old girl was prescribed a 10-fold higher dose of codeine than normal. Upon realizing that the dose was high for a child, the pharmacist dispensing the outpatient medication suggested that the parents give the child only half of the dose. The pharmacist treated the pediatric patient like a "little adult," which resulted in a trip to the intensive care unit for treatment of narcotic-induced respiratory depression. Fortunately, the patient recovered from this medication error (Kozer 2006).

This examples illustrates that although not optimal, caring for pediatric patients does sometimes require extrapolation of adult drug information. Even when this is necessary, keeping in mind the following differences in medication use can enhance the safety of treating pediatric patients.

Dosing
Because of the wide variety of sizes and levels of development in children described in this chapter, pediatric patients need specific dosing based on body weight or BSA.

- The most common approach to dosing pediatric patients is based on their weight: milligram per kilogram per dose (mg/kg/dose) or milligram per kilogram per day (mg/kg/day)—NEVER substitute "d" for dose or day.

- The mg/kg amount can also vary by age. For example, a premature neonate would have captopril dosed at 0.05 mg/kg/dose, whereas a six-year-old child would have captopril dosed at 0.5 mg/kg/dose. Such wide variation in weight-based dosing is a good example of the complexity of dosing pediatric patients. With such complexity, it is safer to consistently refer to appropriate pediatric reference books rather than trying to memorize dosing for each individual drug.

- BSA dosing (mg/m^2/dose) is mostly used to dose chemotherapy or physiologic doses of corticosteroids. BSA is often considered to be a more accurate reflection of body size with regard to drug exposure and elimination. BSA can also be used to extrapolate dosing from adults when no pediatric information is available (Payne 2007). You can calculate BSA by taking the square root of the child's height in centimeters (cm) multiplied by his or her weight in kg, and then dividing by 3,600:

$$\sqrt{(cm \times kg)/3,600} = BSA(M^2)$$

- Some drugs used in pediatric patients are dosed based on pharmacokinetic monitoring. Examples include aminoglycosides, vancomycin, and certain anticonvulsants. The target ranges for peak and trough levels are similar to the ranges used in adults.

- For larger children and adolescents, avoid dosing for weight or BSA when the calculated dose would exceed typical doses (famotidine dosing example: 0.5 mg/kg/dose in a 4 kg patient = 2 mg per dose, but 0.5 mg/kg/dose in an 80 kg patient = ~~40 mg~~ $\longrightarrow$ 20 mg per dose).

- In addition to differences in the dose of medication given to pediatric patients, there can also be differences in the dosing interval. Because children can metabolize medications faster than adults, they may require a more frequent dosing interval. Theophylline is an example of a medication that needs to be dosed more frequently in children than in adults.

- You can find ranges of recommended dosing for pediatric patients in tertiary references such as Lexi-Comp's *Pediatric Dosage Handbook* and the comprehensive online drug reference *Micromedex*. It is important to keep in mind that most of these pediatric dosing ranges have not been validated with clinical trials or dose ranging studies. They are often recommendations that have been derived from case reports, clinical experience, or adult dosing.

- Several disease states require alterations in dosing. Cystic fibrosis is an inherited disorder that results in increased clearance of antibiotics and a need for higher dosing. Certain gastrointestinal disorders require increases in dosing secondary to poor absorption. However, kidney and liver disorders can result in the need for decreased doses because of poor clearance.

- Renal dosing in children is approached in a similar way to how it is approached in adults, with doses and intervals being adjusted based on estimated creatinine clearance (CrCl). Whereas the Cockcroft-Gault equation is typically used in adults, the Schwartz formula is used in pediatric patients. The Schwartz formula gives a CrCl result that is normalized to a normal adult-sized patient, as reflected by the units mL/min/1.73 m^2.

Transitioning to adult dosing can be confusing—when exactly does a "pediatric patient" become an "adult patient"? Different practitioners and different references will give varying opinions. Generally, a pediatric patient is considered to be able to take adult doses when the patient reaches adolescence (age 13 years) or 40 kg. These limits for pediatric dosing do not apply to all patients. For example, adolescents who are very small—such as a 19 kg 15-year-old with cerebral palsy—will still require pediatric dosing. The best approach is to dose patients by weight until their weight-based dose reaches adult doses. In these cases, the patient should be given adult doses with further adjustments based on their clinical condition.

Administration

Not all medications come in dosage forms that are suited to pediatric administration. When altering medications for use in pediatric patients (e.g., compounding liquid preparations, cutting or crushing tablets, or making powder dilutions), you need to consider several things:

- Most medications are manufactured for adults; therefore, children will rarely receive a whole vial, tablet, or unit dose cup of any medication. Obtaining an entire adult dosage form or multiple vials or tablets to administer a pediatric dose should be a red flag for the nurse to double-check the dose.

- Liquids are the ideal oral dosage forms for pediatric patients because many find it difficult—or simply refuse—to swallow solid medications.

- The options for oral dosage forms may be limited due to lack of commercially available liquid dosage forms. Compounded liquids are an option, but the stability of the compounded medications needs to be confirmed before administration. Several published references contain recipes for compounding specialized dosage forms for pediatrics. In addition, pharmacies that provide pediatric services often have a record of recipes that have been used successfully within their institution.

- Chewable tablets are not available for many drugs, but they can be useful for patients older than four years of age. Younger children may not be able to chew and swallow the tablet completely and thus are at risk for choking on the solid dosage form.

- As a general rule, you may *NOT* alter extended-release products due to the risk of dose-dumping with disruption of the timed-release properties. Extended-release products also should not be chewed or given in food that a young patient may chew.

- Capsules are sometimes opened and their contents sprinkled into food for administration to small children. Because some medications have special pH coatings that may require an acidic or basic environment for optimal effect, you should consult drug references or a pharmacist before administering medications mixed in food.

- The osmolality of the final formulation needs to be considered. Osmolality (mOsm/kg) and osmolarity (mOsm/mL) are basically interchangeable terms for the amount of solute in a given amount of liquid (Erstad 2003). The difference is determined by how the concentration was measured (Erstad 2003). Generally, liquid medications are discussed in terms of osmolality, whereas the measure of osmoles in a patient is discussed in terms of osmolarity. Products with high osmolality can cause tissue irritation when administered enterally or parenterally. For enteral nutrition, the American Academy of Pediatrics (AAP) recommends osmolarity limits of 400 mOsm/L, which roughly correlates to an osmolality 450 mOsm/kg (AAP 1976, Jew 1997). Various references identify the osmolarities of certain commonly used drugs, but it can be difficult to find the osmolality of a given drug (Dickerson 1998; Jew 1997). When drug-specific osmolarities cannot be found, the safest approaches are to separate administration of multiple medications as much as possible, dilute medications in free water or continuous feeds as available, and monitor the patient carefully for any new or worsening signs of gastrointestinal irritation. Involvement of a pharmacist is also an option to help enhance the safety and tolerability of liquid oral medications. High osmolality in intravenous (IV) solutions is especially important for patients that do not have central line access. A typical level to stay below is 1,000 mOsm/L. The limits vary per drug and type of access (central versus peripheral) and are dictated by published data as well as prior in-house experience. The risk of hyperosmolar solutions through a peripheral line is not simply venous irritation but also potential loss of the line access.

- Intramuscular (IM) injections may require more volume than can be safely administered into the small muscles of children. Age-specific volumes of IM injections are listed in drug references (Robertson 2005). In addition, many hospitals and pediatric units may have their own unpublished limits based on prior clinical experience and patient tolerance.

- Although more of an issue for neonates, some IV products need to be further diluted to deliver an appropriate, measurable dose.

- You may need to concentrate IV medications so that the patient does not receive too much fluid. Fluid restriction is most important in neonates, infants, patients with cardiac abnormalities, patients with poor kidney function, and patients receiving multiple IV medications.

- You should *NOT* cut transdermal patches into smaller doses for safety reasons. A safe alternative is to cover part of the patch with a bandage to reduce the administered dose.

- Inhaled medications, such as metered dose inhalers and dry powder inhalers, may be difficult for children to use properly. The use of spacers or nebulizers can improve the child's ability to obtain adequate dosing of aerosolized products. In general, you can give equivalent doses of aerosolized medications to children because their lung anatomy and physiology will limit the actual dose received.

- Rectal administration is an option, but it is not preferred unless the patient is unable to take medications orally. Unpredictable absorption, patient discomfort, risk of bleeding or infection in patients with low blood cell counts, and inadequate retention of the suppository or solution are reasons that rectal administration is discouraged.

Monitoring

The wide variety of patient variables, combined with the limited study information on doses and dosage forms used in children, requires a greater role for monitoring drug therapy in this patient population. Recommended dosing ranges are often extrapolated from adult information. Therefore, the actual doses required to reach a therapeutic endpoint in children may be above recommended dosing. Slow, careful titration should guide therapy that is above recommended dosing ranges.

Because pediatric patients handle drugs differently, they may experience exaggerated or unique side effects not seen in adults. Looking at the primary literature for case reports of similar events in children is a good way to identify adverse drug events not commonly reported in tertiary references.

Pharmacokinetic monitoring can provide useful information, but there are limitations to its usefulness in pediatric patients. The increased clearance of antibiotics in some children can make levels seem unreliable. Other children may require higher levels of anticonvulsants than adults do in order to remain seizure-free. Ultimately, the patient's clinical response is more important than a lab value.

Differences in medication safety

Because pediatric patients are at a greater risk for DRPs and require unique methods of medication use, they are also at a greater risk for sustaining serious injury from medication errors. A vital part of caring for pediatric patients involves a systems approach to medication safety:

- Providing services from a satellite that dispenses medication for pediatric patients only

- Standardizing the preparation of high-risk medications such as chemotherapy and drips

- Standardizing doses by weight ranges for wide therapeutic index drugs

- Dispensing medications as the final ordered dose in individual unit dose packaging

- Requiring double-check calculations for high-risk medications such as chemotherapy

- Using computer programs in appropriate situations to reduce human calculation error

- Educating pharmacists, nurses, and physicians with regard to the unique medication safety needs of children

- Improving the order-writing process:
  - Including mg/kg/dose on all weight-based orders
  - Eliminating the use of unsafe abbreviations (See chapter 2 for further discussion of unsafe abbreviations)
  - Proper use of leading and trailing zeros (.1 = 0.1; 1.0 = 1)

Many of these systems approaches to patient safety are formally recommended by the AAP in its policy statement on the prevention of medication errors in the pediatric inpatient setting (AAP 2003).

Chapter 2 | General pediatric medication safety principles

Learning objectives

After reading this chapter, the reader will be able to:

- Identify the "six rights" of safe pediatric high-alert medication administration

- Describe the role that The Joint Commission's National Patient Safety Goals play in pediatric high-alert medication safety initiatives

- Identify the role that error reporting plays in improving pediatric high-alert medication safety

What are high-alert medications?

High-alert medications include medications that are frequently prescribed, are frequently given in error, have a high risk for causing harm when used incorrectly, and, in some cases, have been singled out by safety and regulatory bodies for their potential for causing harm to patients. Concern surrounding pediatric high-alert medications has garnered increased attention from institutions and organizations nationwide. Professional associations, regulatory bodies, and even the news media have all targeted safety, especially medication safety, as a significant problem in today's healthcare system. This increased attention stems from mounting awareness surrounding pediatric patients' unique needs, together with the growing body of literature demonstrating an increased number of errors occurring in the pediatric population (AAP Policy Statement 2003; Alton et al. 2006; Hughes and Edgerton 2005; Levine et al. 2001).

Studies also suggest increased morbidity as a result of medication errors occurring in children compared to adults (AAP Policy Statement 2003; Alton et al. 2006; Hughes and Edgerton 2005; Levine et al. 2001). Current research and education targets a number of general safety principles, all focused on preventing errors related to dosing, dispensing, and administering medications to children.

For a list of the Institute for Safe Medication Practices' (ISMP) list of high-alert medications (for all patient populations), see Figure 2.1.

Figure 2.1   ISMP's list of high-alert medications

 Institute for Safe Medication Practices

ISMP's List of *High-Alert Medications*

High-alert medications are drugs that bear a heightened risk of causing significant patient harm when they are used in error. Although mistakes may or may not be more common with these drugs, the consequences of an error are clearly more devastating to patients. We hope you will use this list to determine which medications require special safeguards to reduce the risk of errors. This may include strategies like improving access to information about these drugs; limiting access to high-alert medications; using auxiliary labels and automated alerts; standardizing the ordering, storage, preparation, and administration of these products; and employing redundancies such as automated or independent double-checks when necessary. (Note: manual independent double-checks are not always the optimal error-reduction strategy and may not be practical for all of the medications on the list).

Classes/Categories of Medications
adrenergic agonists, IV (e.g., epinephrine, phenylephrine, norepinephrine)
adrenergic antagonists, IV (e.g., propranolol, metoprolol, labetalol)
anesthetic agents, general, inhaled and IV (e.g., propofol, ketamine)
antiarrhythmics, IV (e.g., lidocaine, amiodarone)
antithrombotic agents (anticoagulants), including warfarin, low-molecular-weight heparin, IV unfractionated heparin, Factor Xa inhibitors (fondaparinux), direct thrombin inhibitors (e.g., argatroban, lepirudin, bivalirudin), thrombolytics (e.g., alteplase, reteplase, tenecteplase), and glycoprotein IIb/IIIa inhibitors (e.g., eptifibatide)
cardioplegic solutions
chemotherapeutic agents, parenteral and oral
dextrose, hypertonic, 20% or greater
dialysis solutions, peritoneal and hemodialysis
epidural or intrathecal medications
hypoglycemics, oral
inotropic medications, IV (e.g., digoxin, milrinone)
liposomal forms of drugs (e.g., liposomal amphotericin B)
moderate sedation agents, IV (e.g., midazolam)
moderate sedation agents, oral, for children (e.g., chloral hydrate)
narcotics/opiates, IV, transdermal, and oral (including liquid concentrates, immediate and sustained-release formulations)
neuromuscular blocking agents (e.g., succinylcholine, rocuronium, vecuronium)
radiocontrast agents, IV
total parenteral nutrition solutions

Specific Medications
colchicine injection
epoprostenol (Flolan), IV
insulin, subcutaneous and IV
magnesium sulfate injection
methotrexate, oral, non-oncologic use
oxytocin, IV
nitroprusside sodium for injection
potassium chloride for injection concentrate
potassium phosphates injection
promethazine, IV
sodium chloride for injection, hypertonic (greater than 0.9% concentration)
sterile water for injection, inhalation, and irrigation (excluding pour bottles) in containers of 100 mL or more

Background

Based on error reports submitted to the USP-ISMP Medication Errors Reporting Program, reports of harmful errors in the literature, and input from practitioners and safety experts, ISMP created and periodically updates a list of potential high-alert medications. During February-April 2007, 770 practitioners responded to an ISMP survey designed to identify which of these medications were most frequently considered high-alert drugs by individuals and organizations. Further, to assure relevance and completeness, the clinical staff at ISMP, members of our advisory board, and safety experts throughout the US were asked to review the potential list. This list of drugs and drug categories reflects the collective thinking of all who provided input.

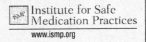 Institute for Safe Medication Practices
www.ismp.org

Source: © Institute for Safe Medication Practices (ISMP), 2007. www.ismp.org. Used with permission.

The sixth "Right"

Safe dosing, dispensing, and administration of pediatric high-alert medications require a multidisciplinary, multisystem approach to medication safety. Although most documented errors occur before a medication is administered to the patient, as is the case in dosing errors or transcription mistakes, nurses play a significant role in pediatric medication safety (Fortescue et al. 2003). Because nurses are the ones who most frequently administer medications to patients, they are often the last layer of protection between a medication error and the potential for serious harm to the patient (Hughes and Edgerton 2005).

The "five Rights" (commonly referred to as the "5 Rs") of safe medication administration are a well-known foundation to most safety programs. When it comes to safe medication administration in children, however, a sixth "Right" must be considered. The right age-appropriate approach to the child, explanations, and administration techniques are crucial considerations when it comes to safe medication administration in children (Bowden and Greenberg 1998). Different sources define the common "Rights" of safe medication administration in various ways. The most common "Rights" and the ones we have focused on throughout this book include the following list.

✓ The RIGHT patient

✓ The RIGHT medication and dose

✓ The RIGHT route

✓ The RIGHT frequency

✓ The RIGHT time

✓ The RIGHT age-appropriate approach, explanation, and administration techniques

The "6 Rs" of safe medication administration are especially important when administering high-alert medications.

Case study

System errors

In 1996, a hospital medication error resulted in the tragic death of a newborn. The error involved the administration of a tenfold overdose of the intramuscular medication penicillin G benzathine by the IV route. As a result, three nurses were indicted on charges of negligent homicide. In the months and years that followed this case, system analyses of the processes involved were performed not only by the hospital and legal teams but also by organizations such as the Institute for Safe Medication Practices (ISMP) and safety organizations nationwide. The ISMP analysis found more than 50 different failures in the systems that allowed this error to develop, remain undetected, and ultimately reach the patient (Smetzer 1998).

1. Based on the preceding information, what two "rights" were not followed?

2. How could this have been prevented?

3. What processes do you have in place in your institution or in your own practice to decrease the chance of such an error occurring?

Although essential, the "6 Rs" alone are not enough when it comes to ensuring pediatric high-alert medication safety. Prior to administering *any* medications to a pediatric patient, the nurse also must confirm the following (Fortescue et al. 2003; Hughes and Edgerton 2005):

✓ Correct patient, using two unique identifiers such as name and medical record number

✓ Patient's current weight, in kilograms (kg)

✓ Whether the weight on the order matches the patient's current weight, in kg

✓ Allergy status

✓ Reason for the medication

✓ Any previous reaction(s) to the medication

✓ The safe dose range for the medication based on the patient's weight and intended use of the medication

✓ Potential side effects

✓ Compatibility related to other medications or IV solutions

National Patient Safety Goals

Although nurses are not responsible for prescribing, transcribing, and dispensing medications, they must be aware of The Joint Commission's National Patient Safety Goals and guidelines that apply to all steps in safe medication administration practices, because often nurses are the final step, or layer, in safe medication administration practices. The Joint Commission's National Patient Safety Goals describe a number of guidelines applicable to accurate prescribing, transcribing, dispensing, and administration of pediatric high-alert medications (The Joint Commission 2007).

Dangerous abbreviations and dosing guidelines

In 2001, The Joint Commission first issued an alert related to an increased number of reported errors associated with misinterpreted medical abbreviations. Since that time, a group of "do not use" abbreviations has been created and the list has been integrated into The Joint Commission surveys. Adhering to this list is considered the minimum an institution must do when it comes to medical abbreviations.

Other groups, such as the Institute for Safe Medication Practices (ISMP), have expanded on The Joint Commission requirement. The ISMP publishes a list of error-prone abbreviations, symbols, and dose designation, which can be found at *www.ismp.org*. Although The Joint Commission recommendations are considered a required element for institutional surveys, organizations are encouraged to incorporate ISMP guidelines as well as other abbreviations found to be potentially hazardous within the organization into organizationwide "do not use" policies.

For additional information about The Joint Commission "do not use" abbreviations, visit *www. jointcommission.org*.

Tips to remember

✓ Know the standardized list of abbreviations, acronyms, symbols, and dose designations that are not to be used throughout the organization.

✓ Write out all instructions rather than using abbreviations

✓ *Do not use* abbreviations of drug names—write them out (e.g., MS could mean morphine sulfate or magnesium sulfate). Do not accept medication orders that have been written using abbreviations.

✓ *Avoid* trade names—use generic medication names instead.

✓ Do not use abbreviations—spell out dosage units

✓ Do not use dose ranges (e.g., "200–400 milligrams every six hours"); make instructions specific (e.g., "200 milligrams every six hours").

✓ *Do not use* a trailing zero to the right of a decimal point to minimize tenfold dosing errors (e.g., use 7 rather than 7.0). *Do use* a zero to the left of a dose less than 1 to minimize the chance of a tenfold errors (e.g., use 0.1 rather than .1).

✓ *Do not use* verbal orders whenever possible. If verbal or telephone orders are necessary, *do not use* abbreviations and spell out the common error words (such as numbers [fifteen versus fifty] and units of measurement [milligrams versus micrograms]); include the dosing weight (10 kg), the weight-based dose (5 mg/kg), the final dose (50 mg), the route, and frequency; and "read back" the transcribed order to the physician or prescriber.

Source: AAP Policy Statement 2003; The Joint Commission 2005.

Many facilities print "do not use" abbreviations at the top of order sheets. Inova Fairfax Hospital for Children prints the following do not use abbreviations:

U, IU, µg, QOD, QID, QD/qd, AU, AS, AD, MS, MS04, MgS04. AZT, Nitro drip

Case study

Telephone orders

Jane is a two-month-old being cared for in the PICU following repair of a congenital heart defect. Jane weighs 4 kg. She is two days postop and her arterial blood gases reflect worsening acidosis. The nurse calls the attending physician and the attending gives the nurse a telephone order for 2 mEq of sodium bicarbonate (4.2% solution 5 mEq/10 ml) IV over two hours. The nurse administers the medication as ordered and repeats the arterial blood gas. Jane's acidosis has worsened. She calls the attending with the follow-up information, and when the attending asks her how much sodium bicarbonate the baby received, the nurse repeats "2 mEq over two hours, just what you ordered." The physician responds with "I didn't say 2 mEq, I said 2 *mEq/kg*." The baby receives an additional dose of sodium bicarbonate as well as a normal saline bolus and her blood gases begin to improve.

1. What went wrong in this interaction between the physician and the nurse?

2. How could this error have been avoided?

Standardization of concentrations

The process of ordering, preparing, and administering continuous medication infusions allows for several opportunities for error. Providing the correct weight-adjusted dose (at an acceptable rate, concentration, and volume) usually requires a multivariable calculation; moreover, a new calculation must be performed whenever the dose is changed.

The need for individualized concentrations makes drip preparation a high-frequency and time-consuming task for the pharmacy. The use of standard drug concentrations eliminates the need to prepare a large number of individualized concentrations, thus decreasing the chance of a high-alert medication error due to individualized continuous medication infusion preparation (Larsen et al. 2005). The Joint Commission forced the hand of many organizations to address this when, by means of the National Patient Safety Goals, it stated that facilities must standardize and limit the number of drug concentrations used by the organization.

See Figure 2.3 for an example of a standard concentration order entry.

Figure 2.3	Standard concentrated drip document

USE BLACK BALLPOINT PEN - PRESS FIRMLY

abcdefghijklmnopqrs Authorization is hereby given to dispense a chemically identical drug (according to hospital formulary) unless otherwise specified.

Order Date & Time	Medication / Infusion Orders	Weight- 1.2 kg	Noted / Time
September 12, 2007 8:48:38 PM	**IV FLUIDS & ELECTROLYTE INFUSIONS**		
September 12, 2007 8:48:38 PM	**DRUG INFUSIONS**		
#1	Dopamine Infusion (0.8 mg/ml) Add 24mg in D5W to make a total drip volume of 30 ml. Infuse at 10 mcg/kg/min which equals 0.9 ml/hour. [Rate in ml/hour = Dose in mcg/kg/min X 0.09]	Dopamine Drip at 0.9 ml/hour	
#2	Fentanyl Infusion (4 mcg/ml) Add 100mcg in D5W to make a total drip volume of 25 ml. Infuse at 1 mcg/kg/hour which equals 0.3 ml/hour. [Rate in ml/hour = Dose in mcg/kg/hour X 0.3]	Fentanyl Drip at 0.3 ml/hour	

Rate (ml/hr) = Dose x Multiplication Factor   Multiplication factor = Wt / Drip Conc x 60 (drips dosed per MINU) = Wt / Drip Conc (for drips dosed per HOUR

(** Note: All infusion rates have been rounded to 2 decimal place. Hence the exact amount of drug delivered may differ very slightly from that ordered.)

Orders entered by Doc, Pager #: 9999   Signature:

PATIENT IDENTIFICATION

abcdefghijklmnopqrs.   Med Rec: 123456789
DOE 2/12/2007   NICU, Room No:

FAIRFAX INOVA HOSPITAL
PHYSICIAN'S ORDERS

TPN 2000, Copyright Marvin Medi-Soft, Inc. 1999

Source: Used with permission from V. Vaidya at TPN2000: Neonatal & Pediatric Software (www.tpn2000.com), Inova Fairfax Hospital for Children / Inova Health System and Fairfax Neonatal Associates (FNA).

Standardization of doses

A hospital or institutional weight-based dosing policy requiring the amount/kg/dose, the patient's weight, and the final amount/dose is an important step in ensuring complete pediatric orders. Similar to the idea of standard concentrations for continuous infusion medications, institution-wide standard weight-based dosing recommendations also improve safety within the pharmacy by minimizing the variations in doses that one pharmacy must prepare for an entire pediatric facility.

Additional safety considerations

In addition to the safety considerations already discussed, there are others that should be followed to ensure patient safety:

Label all medications, medication containers (e.g., syringes, medicine cups, basins), or other solutions on and off the sterile field (The Joint Commission 2007). This includes flush solutions, betadine or other skin prep solutions, medications placed in medicine cups, and of course, any intravenous fluid or medication. Sterile pens and labels are commercially available and frequently used in operating room settings as well as for labeling medications on a sterile field during bedside procedures. *Never* administer an unlabeled, unidentified medication.

Identify and, at a minimum, annually review a list of look-alike/sound-alike drugs used by the organization, and take action to prevent errors involving the interchange of these drugs (The Joint Commission 2007). A classic example is heparin. Heparin is available in a large range of concentrations and the concentration that is appropriate for a neonate is very different from the concentration used for a child or adolescent. Actions that organizations must take include reviewing how medications are stocked, in both the pharmacy and areas accessible to healthcare providers. One approach in a pharmacy is to segregate one item of an infamous sound-alike, look-alike pair to a unique, sound-alike, look-alike drug area. This way, if you are going to pick sulfasalazine, it is not possible to accidentally pick the sulfadiazine that ordinarily might be in the next bin over. The usual bin for sulfadiazine would be labeled with a reminder to obtain the drug from the sound-alike, look-alike area. Over time, experienced pharmacists and healthcare providers may start to recognize a medication by the shape of the container, the color of the cap, or even the font on the label. *Anyone* handling medications must always read the label carefully, and always have a second person double-check and verify high-alert medications before administration (Levine et al. 2001; ISMP).

Common mix-up: Metformin and metronidazole

Flagyl® (metronidazole) and **Glucophage®** (metformin)

Potentially serious mix-ups between metronidazole and metformin have been linked to look-alike packaging (both bulk bottles and unit-dose packages) and selection of the wrong product after entering "MET" as a mnemonic.

What can be done to avoid this potential error?

- Design computer order-entry software to display the entire names of associated products whenever the "MET" stem is used as a mnemonic.

- Use tall man letters for unique letter characters in medication names (e.g., DOPamine and DOBUTamine.

- Stock doses that can not easily be confused. For example, consider stocking metronidazole in only 250 mg tablets (metformin tablets are not available as 250 mg tablets).

Source: www.jointcommission.org.

An example of one hospital pharmacy's collection of look alike-sound alike medications

From The Joint Commission top 10 problem list:

CISplatin (Platinol) vs. CARBOplatin (PARAplatin)

HYDROmorphone vs. morphine

SUfentanil (SUfenta) vs fentanyl

NovoLIN , NovoLOG, NovoLOG mix (all insulins)

LANTUS vs lente (insulins)

Amphotericin LIPID (Ambisome) vs. amphotericin B (non-liposomal)

DOXOrubicin LIPID (Doxil)

PACLItaxel (TaxOL) vs. DOCEtaxel (TaxoTERE)

From Inova problem list:

sulfaDIAzine—sulfaSALAzine

INFLIXimab-RITUXimab

Source: Used with permission from Inova Fairfax Hospital/Inova Fairfax Hospital for Children Pharmacy Department/Inova.

Improve communication among caregivers. Medication safety can be dramatically improved through enhanced communication among caregivers. This includes improved communication with families as well as improved communication among caregivers during transitions and from shift to shift. Make parents a part of the care team. Remember that parents know their child better than anyone. Their observations, assessments, and feedback must be taken into account. If a parent questions a medication or dose, double-check it. Studies have shown that, in these instances, the parent is often right (McKenry and Salerno 2003) and is an important link in patient safety. The shift-to-shift report should include a review of all medications, including scheduled, PRN, and continuous infusions. Take advantage of having two people present to double-check medication schedules as well as all continuous fluid orders, pump rates, and any titration plans.

Accurately and completely reconcile medications across the continuum of care (The Joint Commission 2007). Healthcare organizations must have a process for comparing the patient's current medications with those ordered for the patient while under the organization's care (The Joint Commission 2007). For example, if a child is admitted to an inpatient unit for asthma, the hospital must have a process in place for identifying and documenting *any* medications the child takes at home, not just those related to asthma, as well as new medications that may be started during the child's stay in the hospital.

Parents are often focused on the acute problem, and they may overlook other routine medications. Emergency nurses can give endless examples of families that answered "no" when they were asked in triage whether their child was taking any medications but later responded with "by the way, she also needs (a list of routine medications) at home." Parents must be prompted to recall and identify any medication the child routinely relies on, even those unrelated to the current problem. This process, known as medication reconciliation, will help to ensure that all of the child's healthcare needs are attended to, and it will raise awareness of any possible drug compatibility issues that may arise with the addition of new or different medication regimens.

To reinforce the importance of accuracy in the continuum of care, The Joint Commission also requires that a complete list of the patient's medications be communicated to the next care provider when a patient is referred or transferred to another setting, service, practitioner, or level of care within or outside the organization. The complete list of medications also must be provided to the patient on discharge from the facility (The Joint Commission 2007). Healthcare organizations must have a process in place for seamless communication of medications, from admission through discharge, encompassing everyone involved in caring for the child, including the parents, .

For additional and up to date information about all of The Joint Commission's National Patient Safety Goals, visit The Joint Commission's Web site at *www.jointcommission.org*.

Identifying and reporting errors is critical to safety improvement

If a pediatric medication error or adverse drug event occurs, it is crucial that the event is reported. Institutions have standard processes for reporting errors and adverse events. Without accurate reporting, systems and processes cannot be adapted, fixed, or changed to improve patient safety. It is essential that institutions build safe systems for nurses and healthcare workers to practice within, but if they break down, a safe, nonpunitive process for reporting errors and events must be available. Institutions also must design and have in place processes for honest and timely disclosure to patients and families if an error or adverse event occurs. It is because of accurate error reporting that we are better able to learn from our mistakes, improve our processes, and prevent errors from happening in the future.

Anonymous error reporting

The old adage "we learn from our mistakes" is sometimes painfully true when it comes to high-alert medication safety. For a long time, however, hospitals and other organizations kept error-related information buried, fearing others might learn of mistakes that were made. In the late 1990s, some of the premiere safety organizations, including the ISMP, The Joint Commission, and the Institute of Medicine (IOM), moved to change this and started publishing errors that had been reported or discovered by them (ISMP Historical Timeline). They issued *Medication Safety Alerts, Sentinel Event Reports* and other such tools, alerting healthcare organizations and providers of errors that had occurred and suggesting steps and procedures to minimize the chance of similar mistakes occurring in the future.

Adding to the increased reporting trend, a significant number of organizations have promoted anonymous error reporting and have designed systems for use by their members so that, in the event a mistake occurs, others can learn from it, address safety processes within their own organization, and hopefully prevent the same mistake from occurring in the future. Pediatric-focused quality improvement organizations such as National Association of Children's Hospitals and Related Institutions (NACHRI) and The Vermont Oxford Network (VON) are just two groups using anonymous error reporting to promote improving patient safety processes for those caring for neonates and children of all ages.

When it comes to caring for pediatric patients, there are six "Rights" of safe medication administration. The Joint Commission and other national safety organizations play a significant role in improving patient safety and decreasing pediatric high-alert medication errors. Their recommendations and regulations affect various steps in safe medication administration practices and must be adhered to by all those who care for pediatric patients. In the event, however, that an error or adverse event should occur, it is essential that the event be reported. Error and event reporting ultimately leads to improved safety processes and hopefully minimizes the chance that a similar mistake could happen to another child, another family, and another healthcare provider or providers.

Interested in searching the Internet for more information about pediatric high-alert medication safety? Try the ISMP "Links to Related Sites" at *www.ismp.org/Tools/links.asp.*

**Case
study**

Painful lessons

In 2001, 18-month old Josie King was admitted to The Johns Hopkins Hospital with severe burns received after climbing into a hot bathtub. Weeks passed and Josie was healing well. Josie's family was preparing to bring her home when Josie died unexpectedly of severe dehydration and misused narcotics. Since Josie's death, her family has publicly partnered with Johns Hopkins to improve all aspects of patient safety, both within Johns Hopkins and nationwide. Josie adds an adorable, heart-wrenching face to the devastating effects of medication errors. Josie and her family serve as a reminder of the importance of reporting errors and learning from our mistakes, so that what happened to Josie and her family never happens again.

To learn more about Josie King and the Josie King Foundation, go to: *www.josieking.org*

Chapter 3 | **Technology that improves safety practices**

Learning objectives

After reading this chapter, the reader will be able to:

- Describe the role technology plays in pediatric high-alert medication safety

- Identify at least two recent technological advances found to be effective in preventing pediatric medication errors

New technology

Children pose a special challenge in the medication ordering and delivery process. Dosages must be calculated individually, weights change rapidly, and stock solutions of medications are often available only in adult concentrations and therefore must be diluted for use in children (Fortescue et al. 2003). Recent studies suggest that emerging technologies may prove effective in the prevention of pediatric medication errors and adverse drug events (Fortescue et al. 2003; Larsen et al. 2005). Although computers and other forms of technology aimed at improving patient safety cannot completely eliminate the element of human error, the most effective and proven inventions are created in such a way as to minimize the opportunity for a host of errors to occur. They serve as a sort of checks-and-balances system by guiding users to make the correct choices, and issuing alerts before an error is made (AAP, 2003). Some of these technologies include standardized equipment, computerized systems, preprinted or computer-generated order sheets, computerized physician order entry (CPOE), smart-pump technology, and bar coding. All have their place in improving pediatric high-alert medication safety, yet we must be careful to avoid a false sense of security. Automated technologies are just one piece of the safety puzzle and must be carefully integrated into multilayer medication safety practices.

Case study

Equipment from another unit

The PICU was nearly full with patients and running low on infusion pumps. The nurses knew they were getting a sick baby from the general pediatric floor, so they started calling around looking for additional equipment. The OR found some extra pumps and quickly delivered them to the PICU. The PICU nurse attempted to program the infusion pump for the baby receiving total parenteral nutrition (TPN) by inputting 13.5 mL/hour (volume limit was not preset). The decimal point key on the pump was somewhat worn and difficult to engage. Without realizing it, the nurse programmed a rate of 135 mL/hour. Fortunately, the error was discovered within one hour when the nurse was going off-shift and performed a double-check with the oncoming nurse. The baby's glucose rose to 363, so the rate of infusion for the TPN was decreased for a while and the baby was fine. Standardized equipment, including pediatric volume limits, would have been able to recognize the error before the infusion even began.

1. What other steps may have caught this error earlier?

2. What processes are in place in your institution to minimize the chance of this type of error occurring?

Computerized systems

Computerized systems can check dose and dosage schedules, drug interactions, allergies, and duplicate therapies (AAP Policy Statement 2003). Systems are available to accommodate the prescriber as well as pharmacists. It is important that all parties, including nurses, also have the ability to perform manual double-checks if the system is down. It is also essential that computer programs are designed to minimize the chance for workarounds or override functions, as this decreases the effectiveness of the safety features. The users of computerized systems should be wary of becoming completely dependent on the technology. Double-check processes must remain in place at all levels to ensure accuracy, including for the prescriber, the pharmacy, and the nurse.

Preprinted/computer-generated order sheets

Preprinted/computer-generated order sheets improve high-alert medication safety by prompting the prescriber to identify and include necessary information. Preprinted/computer-generated order sheets should include a space for the child's weight, the dose (e.g., weight-based dose and total dose), old and new allergies, and the prescriber's name, signature, date, and contact number (AAP Policy Statement, 2003). See Figure 3.1 for an example of a preprinted physician order sheet.

Figure 3.1	**Example of standard orders**

☑ = Routine: If not desired, cross off and initial.

☐ = Orders with open box must be checked if desired

INSTRUCTIONS: Unless otherwise specified, authorization is given to dispense a generic equivalent if available on the hospital formulary. Unless specified, all therapeutic interchanges prevail as approved by the facility specific Pharmacy and Therapeutics Committee. **USE BLACK BALLPOINT PEN – PRESS FIRMLY**

PHYSICIANS ORDERS

Infant Immunization Orders: page 1 of 1

Comorbidities: _____

Length: _____ cm;   Weight: _____ gm; Days of Life: _____

Allergies: ☐ No Known Drug Allergies   ☐ No Known Food Allergies

Allergies: _____ (Reaction): _____

Date/Hour	A. MEDICATIONS *(Orders with open box must be checked if desired)*
	1. ☐ Inactivated Polio Vaccine 0.5 mL subcutaneously X 1
	Give on _____ (date)
	(Recommend: standard doses as recommended by AAP)
	2. ☐ Diphtheria / tetanus / acellular pertussis 0.5 mL IM X 1
	Give on _____ (date)
	(Recommend: standard doses as recommended by AAP)
	3. ☐ Haemophilus b conjugate vaccine 0.5 mL IM X 1
	Give on _____ (date)
	(Recommend: standard doses as recommended by AAP)
	4. ☐ Hepatitis B vaccine 0.5 mL IM X 1
	Give on _____ (date)
	(Recommend: standard doses as recommended by AAP)
	5. ☐ Prevnar 0.5 mL IM X 1
	Give on _____ (date)
	(Recommend: standard doses as recommended by AAP)
	6. ☐ Synagis _____ mg IM X 1
	Give on _____ (date)
	(Recommend: 15 mg/kg/dose)
	7. ☐ Acetaminophen _____ mg PO 20 min prior to DtaP and Q4H PRN X 24 H for fever > 100.5 F and/or irritability. Notify MD if temp > 102 and/or excessive irritability.
	(Recommend: 10 to 20 mg/kg/dose Q 4-6 H PRN)
	8. ☐ Parental consent was obtained for the administration of the ordered immunizations on _____ (date).

ANP/FNP/PA/CNM/ACNP/CNP/RN Signature: _____   Date/Time: _____
(All Inova Fairfax Hospital orders AND any orders with controlled substances require VO or TO from physician)

Physician Signature: _____   Date/Time: _____

Printed Physician Name and ID#: _____

PATIENT IDENTIFICATION	**INOVA FAIRFAX HOSPITAL** **INOVA FAIRFAX HOSPITAL FOR CHILDREN** **INFANT IMMUNIZATION ORDERS** **PHYSICIANS ORDERS** Page 1 of 1 CAT #84147 / R5-02 PKGS OF 250

Source: Used with permission from Inova Fairfax Hospital for Children / Inova Health System.

Computerized physician order entry

Computerized physician order entry (CPOE) is a process of electronic entry of physician orders for the treatment of patients under that physician's care. This type of order entry has been around for quite some time, but it is gaining increased attention in recent literature as a successful tool in preventing high-alert medication errors.

Physician orders are communicated through a computer network to the medical staff (nurses, therapists, or other physicians) or to the departments (pharmacy, laboratory, or radiology) responsible for fulfilling the order (Fortescue et al. 2003). Recent studies suggest that CPOE decreases delay in order completion, reduces errors related to handwriting or transcription, allows order entry at the point of care or off-site, and provides error-checking for duplicate or incorrect doses or tests (Fortescue et al. 2003).

Like preprinted/computer-generated order forms, CPOE does allow for some "forced functions" that improve safety among pediatric high-alert medications, such as requiring the patient's weight (in kilograms, or kg), the intended weight-based (mg/kg) and total dose (mg), information on any allergies, alerting the prescriber to compatibility and volume restrictions, and so on. When CPOE is combined with alerts that take into account patient characteristics such as weight, lab variables, and drug interactions from concomitant medications, it is known as CPOE with advanced clinical decision support (ACDS). This is essential to making the most out of the safety benefits that CPOE has to offer. Unfortunately, few CPOE systems have ACDS specific for pediatric patients (Wang 2007). One major limitation of CPOE, however, is that it cannot intervene at the point of administration.

It is well documented that high-alert medication errors often occur in the prescribing process. Most, however, can be stopped when systems such as those described earlier are in place. Nonetheless, patients and care providers are still vulnerable to errors that can occur at the point of administration. That is why it is especially important that nurses—the individuals most often administering pediatric high-alert medications—continue to use careful double-check systems prior to administering *all* pediatric high-alert medications. It is also important that institutions consider technologies aimed at improving the double-check process before high-alert medications are administered to the patient.

Smart-pump technology

Smart-pump technology is an example of a technology that addresses double-check safety systems prior to high-alert medication administration. The use of standard drug concentrations eliminates the need to prepare a large number of individualized concentrations. However, facilities that use standard drug concentrations must then rely on additional reference tools such as dosing charts, which are tables of precalculated values, to reduce the need for calculations (Larsen et al. 2005). In the absence of such charts, nurses and prescribers must learn how to calculate the rate based on the concentration and desired dose. Recently, smart-pump infusion technology has become available. Smart pumps incorporate sophisticated computer technologies for storing drug information (i.e., the drug library), performing calculations, creating unchangeable dosing units once a drug is selected, storing weight limits and clinical advisories, and checking entered information against dosing parameters (Larsen et al. 2005).

Bar coding

Based on the value, utility, and success of bar coding in other industries, healthcare organizations are beginning to implement such programs in efforts to improve medication safety. Bar-coding systems provide another way to attach a unique identifier to each patient. From medication order entry through transcription, dispensing, and administration, all steps of the medication use process can be tracked, tagged, and matched as a form of double-check and verification. Like computerized systems, bar coding is not a surefire answer to high-alert medication safety, especially if its users find convenient workarounds such as the one described in the following case study. But when they are used as they were intended, they can offer the healthcare industry another layer of safety in high-alert medication administration (Topps et al. 2005).

Standardized equipment

One final technology that you can use for pediatric patients throughout the institution is standardized equipment such as infusion pumps and weight scales (AAP Policy Statement 2003). They will improve consistency and accuracy among caregivers and allow for standard safety features such as volume limits, pressure and occlusion alarms, and tubing requirements.

Chapter 4 | Safely preparing, dispensing, and administering medication to kids of all ages

Learning objectives

After reading this chapter, the reader will be able to:

- Identify at least two pharmacy processes that can improve pediatric high-alert medication safety

- Recognize the safety implications of using the correct syringe type for oral and intravenous medications

- Illustrate child-friendly and developmentally friendly techniques that are useful when administering medications to children ranging in age from infancy through adolescence

Safe preparation and dispensing

In Chapter 1, we distinguished pediatric patients from their adult counterparts. There should be no doubt in your mind: Kids are different and need unique, child- and family-focused care. Similarly, nurses and pharmacists caring for pediatric patients have unique needs, especially when it comes to ensuring high-alert medication safety for all pediatric patients.

Dedicated pediatric pharmacy preparation areas improve high-alert medication safety by limiting the possibility of accidental preparation with adult concentrations or solutions. It also allows an institution to design inherent safety features into the product selection, medication preparation processes, and double-check systems to accommodate the unique needs of pediatric patients and pediatric care providers (AAP Policy Statement 2003; Levine et al. 2001).

Unit dose pharmacy preparation is a *must* for pediatric high-alert medications, and it should be a priority for all institutions caring for pediatric patients. Pharmacy unit dosing means that the professionals trained to dispense pediatric medications—pharmacists—are responsible for preparing and dispensing the medication in a ready to use formulation. This includes any reconstituting, mixing, diluting, or other steps that must be taken to prepare the medication for administration to the patient. Unit dosing by a trained pediatric pharmacist is an essential layer of protection in medication safety. In some instances, certain medications, due to their limited stability, must be prepared by nurses at the patient's bedside. Special care must be taken in these situations, as the pharmacist is no longer involved in the double-check process to ensure dosing accuracy, volume reconstitution, and safe medication preparation. It is important that organizations, as well as pediatric nurses, recognize the safety role that a skilled pediatric pharmacist plays and work to minimize the times these individuals are removed from pediatric medication preparation and dispensing processes (AAP Policy Statement 2003; Levine et al. 2001).

Safe administration

The moment of administration is the final layer in pediatric high-alert medication safety. The person most often responsible for this step is the nurse. Therefore, it is crucial that nurses use the many safety layers inherent to safe high-alert medication administration, including adhering to the "six Rs" at all times, accurately integrating available safety technology, and using all double-check systems to ensure patient safety to the best of their ability. Other issues such as cooperation and compliance in the pediatric population, pediatric medication administration systems, and creative ways to prepare and administer medications to children of all ages are universal challenges to all pediatric care providers, and are the essence of the sixth "Right" to safe medication administration in children. Here are recommendations for addressing some of these challenges.

Preventing infections through handwashing

It might seem out of place to discuss handwashing in the context of high-alert medication safety, but in fact, proper handwashing is an essential component to any safety program, including medication safety. Improved adherence to hand hygiene (i.e., handwashing or use of alcohol-based hand rubs) has been shown to reduce healthcare-related infection outbreaks, transmission of antimicrobial-resistant organisms, and overall infection rates (CDC Fact Sheet 2002).

Proper handwashing is necessary before and after any patient contact and prior to handling or preparing medications or intravenous fluids. It is also essential that healthcare providers lead by example while teaching children and families the steps required to perform good handwashing and that they emphasize the importance of handwashing prior to preparing and administering medications at home.

Creative and safe ways to administer medications

Creative and safe ways of administering intravenous and oral medications to children are part of the *art* of being a pediatric nurse.

Experienced pediatric nurses—and parents—have perfected the art of creative oral medication administration. Crushing tablets and dissolving or disguising powdered medication in another solution is a trick that has stood the test of time. It is important, however, to be familiar with any compatibility challenges and to recognize any time-release features of the medication (Hockenberry, M. & Wilson, and D. 2007).

Oral solutions can often be disguised by slightly more appealing flavors. This is a great opportunity to give children some control by letting them choose the flavor from a list of options whenever possible. (Hockenberry, M. & Wilson, D. 2007).

Finally, keep children safe around the equipment used for medication administration. Keep all medications safely locked and out of reach of children, and never leave medication sitting unattended. Infusion pump key pads should be locked so that curious hands don't find their way to it. Remember, kids love to push buttons!

Syringe safety

Syringe safety is unique to neonates, infants, and toddlers because they are the only group of patients to often receive both their intravenous as well as oral medications in syringes (sometimes even the same size syringes). The smallest and sickest pediatric patients also receive their nutrition—namely formula or breast milk—in a syringe as well, only complicating an already complex scenario. The Joint Commission and the Institute for Safe Medication Practices (ISMP) suggest that medical devices should be used only for the purpose for which they were intended. In other words, intravenous syringes should hold only intravenous medications, and oral medications should be prepared in a syringe intended for oral medication administration only. Oral syringes are often distinguished from intravenous syringes by their tip, their color, and their packaging.

The ISMP also directs that not only should devices be used only for the purpose for which they were intended, but also the ends should not fit into devices for which they were not intended (ISMP 2004). For example, you should never use intravenous tubing as feeding tubing. The institution should stock feeding tubes whose ends are incompatible with those of intravenous adapters so that it is impossible to attach the wrong tubing to the wrong syringe. Product selection and eventual storage location are inherent safety layers that, if not followed, could have devastating outcomes. Finally, remember to discard the cap from any oral syringe in the proper place. Aspiration of caps left at a child's bedside are a real safety concern.

The sixth "Right" in safe medication administration to children

Remember the sixth "Right" when administering to children: the right age-appropriate approach, explanation, and administration techniques. All "Rights" are essential to safe medication practice, but the sixth plays a special role in ensuring accurate medication administration while supporting the child's stage of development and the family's role in medication administration and compliance.

The following brief lists of helpful hints may be useful when administering medications to children of all ages.

Infants

- ✓ Involve the parents. It is important to teach parents or caregivers how to administer medications so that they are successful once they are at home.

- ✓ Hold the infant upright. Avoid laying a baby down flat, and never hold a baby down forcefully during medication administration. This is a mistake that well-intentioned parents sometimes make, and it reinforces why teaching them and involving them early is so important.

- ✓ Medications that are not bitter can be pulled up in an oral syringe (never use IV syringes for PO medications). Slowly instill small amounts of the medication into the side of the infant's mouth. Allow the infant to swallow the medication by sucking. Gently stroke the infant's cheek to encourage sucking. Take your time, and encourage parents to do the same. Hurrying could result in the infant choking or spitting the medication out without swallowing first.

- ✓ Bitter medications, such as liquid vitamins, may need to be mixed with a small amount of formula or breast milk. Use as little of the feeding as possible to help disguise the taste of the medication, and then fill the bottle with the rest of the feeding. Avoid putting medications into an entire feeding. If the baby does not finish the bottle, it will be impossible to know how much of the medication he or she received.

✓ If the medication is an injection, take the infant to a different place, such as a treatment room. This allows the infant's room and crib to remain a safe place, where the infant does not need to worry about potentially painful procedures.

✓ Use developmentally friendly positioning for potentially painful procedures such as starting an IV or injections. You can swaddle a young infant, and wrap an older infant in a sheet or large blanket, leaving only the necessary extremity available (this keeps the limbs contained and provides comfort) and held by another care provider.

✓ Oral sucrose solutions, combined with non-nutritive sucking, have been found to decrease pain in infants younger than two months of age during short procedures, including IV insertion and and subcutaneous or intramuscular injections.

Source: *Bowden and Smith-Greenberg 1998; Harder 2002; Hockenberry, M. & Wilson, D., 2007; Lefrak et al. 2006; McKenry and Salerno 2003.*

Case study

Acetaminophen to an infant

A six-month-old named Maria presents in the ER with a fever of 102°F/38.9°C. The doctor orders oral (liquid) acetaminophen to be given prior to the patient's exam.

1. What additional information do you need about Maria before giving this medication?

2. What additional information do you need to make this order complete and accurate?

3. How would you prepare Maria and her parent(s) for the medication administration?

4. What methods would you use for successful oral medication administration for this six-month-old?

Preschool

✓ Involve the parents. It is important to teach parents or caregivers how to administer medications so that they are successful once they are at home.

✓ Preschool-age children want to know "*why*". Use very short, concrete explanations.

✓ Prepare the child prior to any procedure, such as starting an IV or any sort of injection. Puppets, dolls, or drawings may be helpful during preparation.

✓ Provide a distraction, especially during painful interventions. Bubbles, colored lights, stickers, and storytelling are all helpful with preschool-age children.

✓ Tell preschool-age children what you are going to do and what you need them to do.

✓ Give them a job, such as holding the bandage or holding the juice.

✓ Preschool-age children like to be independent, so promote independence whenever possible. Let them hold the medicine. Let them take their own medicine, but be sure to supervise their efforts.

✓ Give them "positive" or realistic choices. (If it's okay to take a medication before or after a meal, give them the choice. If it's okay to take it with juice or milk, give them a choice. If the medication is an injection, let them choose the right leg or the left leg.) For things that are not optional, do not give them choices. Avoid saying things such as "It's time to take your medicine, okay?" Instead, try "It's time to take your medicine. Do you want to take it with apple juice or orange juice?"

✓ Avoid bribing or, worse yet, threatening a child to take his or her medicine. Bribes, such as "If you take your medicine I will give you a sticker," don't work because taking the medicine is not a choice. Threats, such as "If you don't take your medicine, you can't watch TV," don't work either, because again, taking the medicine isn't a choice.

✓ Never call medicine "candy" or "a treat." Call it what it is: medicine.

✓ Some pills can be crushed and mixed with food such as applesauce, gelatin, pudding, and so on. Make sure that medication can indeed be crushed (enteric coated pills, for example, cannot be crushed). If you are mixing medicine in food, *tell children* that their medicine is in the food (and better yet, let them choose what type of food it will be mixed in). This builds trust between you and them and builds trust in their environment. Mix medications in a small amount of food so that the child is sure to get the entire dose.

✓ If the medication is an injection, take the child to a different place, such as a treatment room. This allows the child's room and bed to remain a safe place, where the child does not need to worry about potentially painful procedures.

✓ *Never* tell a child something isn't going to hurt if there is a chance it will.

✓ Topical anesthetics are helpful for minimizing injection pain.

✓ IM or subcutaneous (SQ) injections should be pushed slowly. The idea of "getting it over quickly" isn't always best for injections, because in many cases, the solution may be painful as it enters the muscle or subcutaneous area, and a slower injection helps decrease the pain.

✓ If the child is not cooperative, despite your best efforts, medication administration may need to be a two-person procedure. Use developmentally friendly positioning methods for holding the child, such as sitting him or her on your lap facing away from you. Give the child a hug by wrapping your arms around his or her arms and holding the child gently, but firmly, against you. Have the second person stand in front of the child, administering the medication. This is a good way to secure a child prior to any injection medications.

✓ Even the most cooperative child will need developmentally friendly positioning methods before an injection or when starting IVs.

✓ After the child has taken the medication or the medication has been successfully administered, praise the child. Remember to use words such as "All done" to let the child know the procedure is complete.

✓ Simple rewards, such as stickers or colorful bandages, work well with preschool-age patients.

Source: *Bowden and Smith-Greenberg 1998; Harder 2002; Hockenberry, M. & Wilson, D., 2007; McKenry and Salerno 2003.*

Case study

Preschool medicine

Sarah, a four-year-old, is hospitalized for appendicitis. She is one-day post-appendectomy and is receiving IV fluids, IV antibiotics, and PRN pain medication. It is time for her third dose of IV ampicillin. Prior to administering Sarah's medication:

1. What additional information do you need about her?

2. What additional information do you need to know about the ampicillin order?

3. How should you prepare her for the medication administration?

4. What methods would you use for successful IV medication administration to a four-year-old?

Source: *Bowden and Smith-Greenberg 1998; Harder 2002; McKenry and Salerno 2003.*

School age

✓ Involve the parents. It is important to teach parents or caregivers how to administer medications so that they are successful once they are at home.

✓ Many of the same techniques suggested for preschool-age children are also appropriate for older school-age children.

✓ Explain the reason for the medication using concrete words that the child will understand.

✓ Give school-age children positive or realistic choices.

✓ Give school-age children as much independence as possible.

✓ Educate children with chronic illnesses about their medications, using language and explanations they can understand. This will help them to begin to develop a sense of responsibility for their health and their medications.

✓ Prepare the child for any procedures related to medication administration. School-age children can begin to understand concepts such as guided imagery and relaxation techniques.

Source: *Bowden and Smith-Greenberg 1998; Harder 2002; Hockenberry, M. & Wilson, D., 2007; McKenry and Salerno 2003.*

Case study

School-age injection preparation

Connor is an eight-year-old newly diagnosed with diabetes. His evening insulin dose is due, and you have also been asked to begin insulin injection teaching with Connor and his dad.

1. How would you prepare Connor for the insulin administration?

2. What methods would you use for successful SQ injections in an eight-year-old?

3. How would you begin teaching Connor and his Dad to perform his injections at home?

Adolescence

✓ Involve the parents. It is important to teach parents or caregivers how to administer medications so that they are successful once they are at home and so that they can properly supervise their adolescent child and promote their independence.

✓ Many of the same techniques suggested for preschool and school-age children are also appropriate for adolescents.

✓ Be alert that children this age may start to hide their medication and pretend they have taken it.

✓ Use honest, factual explanations.

✓ Allow for privacy. Ask the adolescent whether his or her parent(s) should step out during procedures or whether he or she prefers that they stay.

✓ Adolescents are capable of using coping techniques, such as guided imagery and relaxation techniques.

✓ Encourage the use of topical anesthetics for potentially painful procedures.

Source: *Bowden and Smith-Greenberg 1998; Harder 2002; Hockenberry, M. & Wilson, D., 2007; McKenry and Salerno 2003.*

Case study

Adolescent education

Ally, a 16-year-old, is admitted to your unit with increased seizure activity. Ally has a history of seizures and takes routine seizure medication. A new oral medication is being added to Ally's regimen, and she is due for her first dose.

1. How would you prepare Ally for the new medication?

2. What methods would you use for successful oral medication administration for a 16-year-old?

Ensuring compliance

Pediatric medication compliance is a twofold challenge. Neonates, infants, and young children must rely on their parent(s) or caregivers to administer their medications, especially outside a hospital setting. The adult administering the medication must understand why it is being prescribed, how often it must be administered, any potential side effects, and how to measure and administer the medication to the child. It is essential that healthcare providers involve parents and caregivers in the medication process from the very beginning and educate them about the medication their child is being prescribed.

Oral medications can often be difficult to administer to a small child. It is essential that the parent(s) or caregivers understand the importance of getting the child to take the medication, and to do so, nurses must teach them proper methods and helpful hints. Nurses and healthcare providers must also appreciate the cost of medications and the burden that places on some families. If a family does not have prescription health coverage, the family may not refill prescriptions in a timely fashion or may try to stretch medications out beyond their prescribed schedule in an attempt to make them last longer. This is a crucial problem with no easy solutions, but one that today's pediatric healthcare providers must recognize.

As children grow, they seek independence in all aspects of their lives, including their own healthcare. Parents, care providers, and healthcare professionals must recognize this and work with children to support their independence while facilitating their healthcare needs. Medication calendars and contracts are just two ways families and healthcare providers can work together to promote independence as well as medication compliance (Bowden and Smith-Greenberg 1998; Hockenberry, M. & Wilson, D., 2007).

Additional pediatric medication administration safety tips:

✓ Take a careful drug allergy history. Make sure that it is clearly marked on the patient's ID, in the medical record, and in the pharmacy system.

✓ Know the medication you are giving. Do not rely on your memory or on the memory of others. Look it up if you have any questions or are unsure.

✓ Have a pediatric medication reference available wherever medications are prepared and administered. Consult the pharmacy with any questions related to pediatric medication orders, preparation, and administration.

✓ Calculate with confidence. Use a calculator. Double-check calculations with a second nurse.

✓ Minimize distractions during medication preparation.

✓ Document all medications in a timely manner. Do not rely on your memory at the end of the shift. Remember, if it isn't documented, *it wasn't given.* Not documenting could result in a double dose.

✓ Be aware of drug incompatibilities with other medications or intravenous fluids.

✓ Record IV amounts used to deliver IV medications in the intake and output record. Accurate intake and output is especially important in the pediatric population.

Keep kids safe: *Before* medication administration

✓ Confirm that you are working with the correct patient prior to performing any procedure or administering medication using *two* (2) unique identifiers (e.g., name, medical record number, bar code) (The Joint Commission 2007).

✓ Know the child's current weight in kilograms (kg). Do not rely on a parent's memory. If necessary, weigh the child prior to ordering the medications to ensure accuracy.

✓ Know the child's allergy information, including food and medication reactions.

✓ Adhere to the "six Rights" of safe medication administration for children (Bowden and Greenberg 1998).

✓ Know the medication you are administering. It is neither acceptable nor defensible to give a medication to a patient of any age without knowing:

  – Why it is being prescribed

  – How it works (the mechanism of action)

  – The correct dose, including concentration

  – A safe administration route and rate

  – Compatibility with other medications or treatment regimens

  – Expected effect as well as potential side effects

✓ Perform independent double-checks of all high-alert medications prior to administration, programming or adjusting pump doses or rates, and during any handoff or transfer of care (ISMP 2003).

✓ Review medication orders and treatment plans at any handoff, including at change of shift, at change of caregiver, and any time a child is transferred from one level of care to another, including discharge home (The Joint Commission, NPSG 2007).

Keep kids safe: *During* medication administration

✓ Perform independent double-checks of all high-alert medications prior to administering, setting, or adjusting pump doses or rates, and during any handoff or transfer of care (ISMP, March 2003)

✓ Clearly label all medication and flush solutions (The Joint Commission, NPSG 2007)

✓ Clearly label all continuous infusion bags or syringes (The Joint Commission, NPSG 2007)

✓ Ensure that all infusion lines are clearly marked, including at connection ports closest to the patient

✓ Avoid infusing intermittent, IV-push, or piggyback medications through lines containing continuous infusion medications, as this could result in unintended surges or boluses of the continuous infusion

✓ Use different syringe pumps for epidural, feeding, and intravenous infusions

Keep kids safe: Make them partners in safety

✓ Teach children who are old enough and healthy enough to participate in their care to verify the dose when taking medication that is given to them, adding another layer of safety through double-checks to the administration process. Also teach them about how the medication works, the potential side effects, and the prescribed schedule (Hockenberry, M. & Wilson, D., 2007; Levine, et al., 2001).

✓ Provide parents or caregivers with frequent updates regarding the plan of care for their critically ill or recovering child and involve them in as many decisions as possible.

✓ Instruct families on the importance of compliance with routine follow-up visits for necessary laboratory data, medication titration, and general health assessment.

Keep kids safe: Apply the sixth "Right"

✓ Teach children and their parent(s) or caregivers, using rules of the sixth "Right," why they are receiving the medication prescribed for them, how it works, any potential side effects to be alert to, and their role and responsibilities during the medication infusion (Hughes and Edgerton 2005; Bowden and Greenberg 1998; Hockenberry, M. & Wilson, D., 2007).

✓ Children requiring treatment with high-alert medications will likely require frequent blood draws to monitor laboratory data and therapeutic effect. Promote age-appropriate, child-friendly, and developmentally focused techniques when providing comfort during blood draws or any potentially painful or scary procedure (Bowden and Greenberg 1998: Hockenberry, M. & Wilson, D., 2007).

✓ Supportive interventions include topical anesthetics, developmentally friendly containment, distraction (bubbles, storytelling, puppets, colorful lights, etc.), imagery, relaxation, and other techniques appropriate for the child's age, developmental level, and acuity (Bowden and Greenberg 1998; Hockenberry, M. & Wilson, D., 2007).

Teach parents how to support their child. They may be so focused on their child's illness or interventions that they overlook the simple things they can do to comfort their child. Give them simple direction. Make them a part of the team.

✓ Even the most acutely ill neonates, infants, toddlers, children, and adolescents need age-appropriate, developmentally friendly, family-focused care to help them heal and keep them safe.

Chapter 5 | # Anticoagulation medications

Learning objectives

After reading this chapter, the reader will be able to:

- Recognize why anticoagulant medications are considered pediatric high-alert medications

- Describe the anticoagulant medications most commonly used in pediatric patients

- Identify at least three ways to prevent errors when administering anticoagulant medications to pediatric patients

Why are anticoagulant medications identified as pediatric high-alert medications?

The Institute for Safe Medication Practices (ISMP), along with The Joint Commission, has identified anticoagulant medications as a group of substances that pose significant risk of causing devastating and often fatal harm when used in error (Taketomo, et al., 2005). Challenges such as look-alike and sound-alike names and packaging, multifaceted calculations, and complex titrating regimens signify just some of the intricate issues underscoring anticoagulants as a high-alert group of medications.

The most important reason that anticoagulants are high-risk medications is their narrow therapeutic index and potential to cause significant bleeding. As further evidence of their high potential for significant adverse events and medication errors, The Joint Commission has recently identified reduction in the likelihood of patient harm from anticoagulants as one of its new patient safety goals for 2008 (The Joint Commission 2007).

There is a complex interplay of substances in the body which—under normal conditions—maintain a fine balance between clot formation (coagulation) and bleeding (anticoagulation). When there is a shift in that balance, the body is at risk for either thrombosis or hemorrhage, both of which can be fatal. You can use a number of medications to alter this complex interplay of substances and shift the balance in either direction. This chapter will focus on medications that shift the balance toward anticoagulation.

Therapeutic options

The term *anticoagulant* is often broadly applied to all medications that increase the fluidity of the blood. However, the more appropriate umbrella term for medications that increase the fluidity of the blood is antithrombotic (AHFS 2007). There are a number of different classifications of antithrombotics, the largest of which is the anticoagulants.

Heparin and the related low molecular weight heparin enoxaparin are both common anticoagulants used in the inpatient setting. When longer-term, outpatient anticoagulation is needed, warfarin is typically the preferred agent, although enoxaparin can be used as well. When patients cannot take heparin due to a condition called heparin-induced thrombocytopenia (HIT), anticoagulation is achieved with direct thrombin inhibitors such as argatroban and lepirudin.

Antiplatelet agents are not frequently used in pediatric patients, but when they are, aspirin and abciximab are the most common choices. Lastly, thrombolytic drugs such as alteplase (tPA) are very powerful agents for lysing clots that have already formed.

Who is at risk?

Thromboembolism and the need for anticoagulant therapy was historically less of a concern in children than in adults. However, the advance of tertiary care pediatrics has led to survival of more severely ill patients—patients who are at high risk for thromboembolism and often require anticoagulant therapy for prevention or treatment of thromboembolism (Monagle et al. 2004).

It is reported that more than 80% of thromboembolic events in children occur in the setting of severe illness (Schneppenheim 2006). Other estimates indicate that 30% of children with venous or arterial thrombotic events have underlying cardiac disorders (Monagle 2004). Overall, the risk of thromboembolic events in pediatric patients is highest in the neonatal period and in postpubertal adolescents (Schneppenheim 2006).

Pediatric considerations

A number of differences in pediatric patients not only affect how they are treated with anticoagulants but also increase their risk for adverse effects.

Epidemiology

In contrast to adults, children are more likely to have proximal vein thrombosis—most likely due to central venous access—than distal venous thrombosis. Arterial thrombosis is less common than venous thrombosis in children (Monagle 2004).

Physiology

The coagulation system in neonates is immature. For example, the ability of a neonate to generate thrombin—a clotting factor essential to coagulation—is delayed and decreased compared to adults (Ronghe 2003, Monagle et al 2004). This difference results in clotting times in untreated children that are comparable to clotting times in adults on therapeutic doses of heparin. In a sense, newborns already exist in a state of anticoagulation. In addition to thrombin, a number of other coagulation factors and inhibitors are decreased in young children.

Changes in the maturation of the coagulation system are not limited to neonates and young children. Differences in the vasculature and coagulation system in adolescents may predispose them to disease-state and therapeutic risks that are unique to those in adults (Monagle 2004). In addition, the activated partial thromboplastin time (aPTT)—a measure of the time it takes the blood to clot—can be longer in neonates or shorter in children depending on the clinical situation (Lexi-Comp 2006). Many pediatricians and pediatric subspecialists make do with the often inaccurate aPTT by monitoring the patient clinically.

Pharmacokinetics

Age-related differences in absorption, distribution, metabolism, and excretion affect the dosing and risk potential of anticoagulants. Oral anticoagulants may be absorbed differently in infants and young children due to an immature or non-functioning GI tract.

Heparin distributes into the fluid compartments of the body. Because water is a higher percentage of body weight compared to adults, there is a greater volume of fluid for the heparin to distribute into in a pediatric patient. This higher volume of distribution in infants and younger children may require higher doses of heparin to achieve the same effect as older patients. This difference in volume of distribution can also lead to a faster clearance of the drug (Monagle et al 2004).

Drug formulations

Anticoagulant therapies used in pediatric patients must rely on customization and preparation from adult dosage forms. Not only is this an inconvenience, but it also can lead to dosing errors in small children.

Drug indications

Due to the low incidence of thrombosis in children, very little clinical trial data is available to guide therapeutic use of anticoagulants in pediatric patients. Therefore, most anticoagulant therapies are being used "off-label" based on information extrapolated from adults.

Medical management

A major limitation to dosing heparin is that there is no therapeutic range specific to children. A dosing nomogram has been published for pediatric patients, but this is based on achieving adult-specific therapeutic ranges. Similar to unfractionated heparin, an enoxaparin dosing nomogram has been published for pediatric patients. There is also a nomogram for warfarin dosing adjustments in pediatric patients; however, the ranges are extrapolated from adult values (Ronghe 2003).

Differences in the medical care of pediatric patients can affect the use of anticoagulants. For example, frequent sedation of children for procedures can limit the ability to diagnose and evaluate thromboembolism. In addition, venous access may be limited in children and may affect the ability to administer and monitor anticoagulation therapy (Monagle 2004).

Compliance

The limited knowledge and increased fear common in pediatric patients also may prove to be a barrier to diagnosis and treatment of thromboembolic disorders, especially when intravenous or subcutaneous dosage forms are needed.

Compliance is particularly a problem when twice-daily subcutaneous injections of enoxaparin are needed for longer-term anticoagulation. Not only are two shots per day troublesome for the child, but the preparation of the correct dose can be troublesome for the parents. The smallest pre-manufactured enoxaparin syringe size is 30 mg/0.3 mL and some infants may require doses that are less than 10 milligrams. This means that the stock solution will need to be diluted and drawn up into a separate syringe for administration. This additional mixing and calculating in the home environment can lead to significant errors. Furthermore, due to stability concerns and limited ability to prepare parenteral dosage forms, most outpatient pharmacies will not prepare these syringes in advance for the patient.

Oral dosing has limitations as well. Warfarin is often prescribed in different strengths on different days in order to keep the blood levels within a narrow therapeutic window. The significant food interactions and restrictions with warfarin also may make compliance difficult.

Unfractionated heparin

Drug-specific information related to unfractionated heparin includes:

- Using "U" or "u" instead of the term *Units* can lead to fatal overdoses.

- Patients should always be followed clinically because aPTT monitoring may not correlate well with actual anticoagulation.

- Heparin is manufactured in a number of concentrations (2, 10, 40, 50, 100, 1,000, 2,000, 2,500, 5,000, 10,000 and 20,000 units/mL) that often come in similar-looking vials. Selection of the wrong concentration when preparing or administering heparin doses can be fatal.

Nursing implications

Multiple concentrations, varying uses, and the challenge of titrating to just the right therapeutic dose for different ages, sizes, and disease processes are just some of the challenges to consider when safely administering heparin to children. Take a look at the "keep kids safe" section in chapter 4 for tips and safety pointers of all high-alert medication.

Administration and safety considerations

- ✓ Make certain the correct heparin concentration is used (Young & Mangum 2007)

- ✓ Heparin lock flush solution is intended to maintain patency of IV devices and is not to be used for anticoagulation therapy (Taketomo, et al., 2005).

- ✓ *Always* double-check the ordered dose against the vial (the concentration) and against the solution that is drawn into the syringe if using for an IV patency flush solution.

- ✓ Consider using normal saline to flush peripheral IV lines instead of heparin-lock solution (IHI).

- ✓ Store saline flush solution separately from heparin solutions (IHI).

- ✓ Consider using normal saline solution bags instead of heparin solutions, as saline is equally good for flushing blood and medications through arterial lines, and it poses minimal risk of causing adverse drug events (IHI).

✓ If heparin solutions are used for any central lines, the pharmacy should add the heparin solution during preparation. Devise systems that require intravenous fluids containing heparin to be ordered by the physician and prepared by the pharmacy only.

✓ Continuous IV infusion of heparin is preferred over intermittent injections (Taketomo, et al., 2005).

✓ Never administer other medications, especially IV-push medications, through a continuous heparin infusion line.

✓ Keep protamine sulfate on hand in the event of an adverse event (Young & Mangum, 2007)

✓ Keep the key pad on the continuous infusion pump locked at all times to minimize the chance of a curious child accidentally changing the rate by pushing the buttons on the key pad.

✓ Children requiring continuous heparin infusions will need frequent blood draws to monitor aPTT and other labs, especially during early use of the medication to ensure a therapeutic level. Promote child-friendly and developmentally friendly techniques when providing comfort during blood draws or when restarting an IV. Additional information about child-friendly and developmentally appropriate techniques for providing comfort during potentally painful procedures can be found in Chapter 4.

Monitoring

✓ Therapeutic use of heparin requires additional attention when administered as a continuous infusion. Monitor platelet counts, signs of bleeding, hemoglobin, hematocrit, and aPTT (Taketomo, et al., 2005).

✓ If intermittent injections are used, follow aPTT three and a half to five hours after IV injection (Taketomo, et al., 2005).

✓ The aPTT can be longer in neonates or shorter in children depending on the clinical situation. Many pediatricians and pediatric subspecialists make do with the often inaccurate aPTT by monitoring the patient clinically.

✓ Laboratory data for a patient receiving heparin therapy is considered critical. Verify results as soon as possible.

Patient and family education highlights

✓ Children receiving anticoagulation therapy are more prone to bruising. This can be very challenging, especially in active children. Educate parents of this risk, and support play and activity that are developmentally appropriate with minimal risk of impact or potential injury.

✓ Hospitalized children requiring continuous heparin infusions will likely be transitioned to a low molecular weight heparin (LMWH) product prior to discharge if continued anticoagulation is necessary. Begin to prepare the parent and child, if appropriate, for this transition using written teaching information and hands-on practice using mannequins or other injection teaching devices.

✓ See the section "Low molecular weight heparins (LMWH)," later in this chapter, for additional information about teaching children and families to perform injections at home.

Case study

Heparin overdose in the NICU

A fatal error involving heparin received national attention in the fall of 2006. Six babies in a NICU received 1,000 times the dose of heparin that they should have received. Three infant deaths resulted when the higher concentration of heparin sodium injection 10,000 units/mL was inadvertently administered instead of the lower concentration of Hep-Lock U/P 10 units/mL. According to reports, the NICU stocked only one dosage of heparin to keep infants' IV lines open. An experienced pharmacy tech mistakenly took the wrong dosage from inventory (both vials have shades of blue labeling and are similar in size and font) and stocked it in the cabinet. The nurses, who were accustomed to only one dose of heparin being available on the unit, administered the wrong dosage.

1. What types of processes or systems could have prevented this error?

2. What is in place in your institution to keep high-alert medication errors such as this from occurring?

For more information about this story, visit the ISMP Web site at *www.ismp.org*.

Low molecular weight heparins

One significant drawback to LMWH is the lack of a true antidote. Protamine does not completely reverse the anticoagulant activity of LMWH as it does for unfractionated heparin. In combination with the longer half-life, this makes dosing for invasive procedures more difficult. In children, it is recommended that two doses of LMWH be held before invasive procedures.

Even within the LMWH class, different methods of depolymerization lead to different-size molecules that result in unique properties for each drug. Therefore, carefully consider the differences between commercially available LMWH products when starting or changing therapy in pediatric patients. Currently, enoxaparin is the LMWH product that has the most experience in the pediatric population.

Nursing implications

Similar to heparin administration, the safety challenges surrounding LMWH administration reflect the wide range of ages for which it is used, the often challenging volumes needed for accurate dosing in the smallest patients, and the challenge of administering primarily subcutaneous injections to children of all ages.

Take a look at the general tips in the "keep kids safe" section of chapter 4.

Administration and safety considerations

✓ LMWH (enoxaparin) is administered using SQ injection only. *Do not* administer intramuscularly (IM) or IV (Taketomo, et al., 2005).

✓ Do not rub SQ injection site after administration, as bruising may result (Taketomo, et al., 2005).

✓ Repeated administration through subcutaneous ports may lead to local thrombosis

✓ SQ catheter systems are available. Once they are inserted, the child or parent infuses the medication via a port instead of via daily injections. The SQ catheter must be routinely rotated.

✓ Topical anesthetics (e.g., lidocaine), ice, or a cold pack applied to the injection site prior to injection may be helpful in decreasing the pain and anxiety of daily or routine SQ injections for children of all ages. (Hockenberry, M. & Wilson, D., 2007).

✓ Rotate sites regularly; keep track of injection sites using a diagram or log, and teach the child and family to do the same once they start to perform injections on their own.

✓ Dosing and pharmacokinetics of LMWHs and unfractionated heparin are different

✓ Dosing and pharmacokinetics of the various LMWHs are different

✓ Some LMWHs are dosed in terms of Units, whereas others are dosed in terms of milligrams

✓ Enoxaparin should be withheld (at least two hours) and antifactor Xa should be determined, if possible, prior to lumbar or epidural procedures (Taketomo, et al., 2005).

✓ Children requiring LMWH injections will need frequent blood draws to monitor laboratory data, especially during early use of the medication to ensure a therapeutic level. Promote child-friendly and developmentally appropriate techniques when providing comfort during blood draws. Additional information about child-friendly and developmentally appropriate techniques can be found in Chapter 9.

Monitoring

Even though LMWHs have a more stable pharmacokinetic profile that limits the need for consistent monitoring in adults, children still require frequent monitoring due to increased risk factors for significant bleeding and the need for frequent adjustment of weight-based dosing. Check antifactor Xa levels four hours after the initial dose and after any dose changes. Once a patient has reached a stable therapeutic range (generally 0.5–1 units/mL) for two consecutive days, confirmation of the therapeutic range can be limited to once monthly monitoring provided there are no dose changes:

✓ Laboratory data related to LMWH is considered critical. Verify results as soon as possible.

✓ Antifactor Xa level assays are different for heparin and LMWHs; make sure the correct assay is used

✓ Lack of pediatric formulations of enoxaparin can result in difficulty preparing the appropriate dose for small patients

✓ Monitor CBC with platelets, stool occult blood tests (Taketomo, et al., 2005).

✓ Consider bone density studies in infants and children with long-term use (Taketomo, et al., 2005).

✓ Be aware of potential drug interactions: Anticoagulants, thrombolytic agents, and platelet inhibitors may increase the risk of bleeding (Taketomo, et al., 2005).

✓ Patients with poor renal function should not receive LMWHs (Taketomo, et al., 2005).

Patient and family education highlights

✓ Teaching parents to give young children a routine injection can be challenging, as is teaching school-age and adolescent children to perform their own injections. Start early—this is not something that can wait until the day the patient is scheduled to go home.

✓ Early instruction should include written information, demonstration, and the opportunity to learn injection techniques on a mannequin or other teaching device. If a teaching doll is unavailable, simple tools such as a ball of clay can help to replicate the feel of performing an SQ injection. (Hockenberry, M. & Wilson, D., 2007).

✓ Provide the child and family with adequate practice drawing up the correct volume in the syringe. SQ injections are usually of a very small volume. Reinforce the importance of accuracy and precision, and again, provide plenty of time to practice.

✓ Provide consistent, positive feedback to the entire family during the education process.

✓ Offer parents suggestions and tips related to how best to provide comfort measures and distraction techniques, and offer children positive feedback during and after injections (Hockenberry, M. & Wilson, D., 2007).

✓ Help children and parents to develop a map or calendar to track the rotation of injection sites.

Educating parents

Tommy is a three-month-old hospitalized in the PICU for severe gastrointestinal bleeding and treatment of a rare esophageal varices rupture. During
his treatment, Tommy underwent a procedure to have a coil placed in the
bleeding vessels. Following the procedure, he was started on a continuous
heparin drip to maintain a stable anticoagulation state. Tommy has recovered
from the procedure, and his family is preparing to take him home from the
hospital. His parents have been told that Tommy will require daily injections
of enoxaparin until he is at least six months of age.

1. Describe the teaching steps necessary to prepare Tommy's family to
   perform his injections.

2. How would you suggest that Tommy's family comfort him during these
   injections?

Warfarin

The half-life of warfarin is long at 36–42 hours, but more important is the half-life of the clotting factors
that warfarin inhibits. Factor VII has the shortest half-life at six hours, so the initial anticoagulant effects
can be seen 8–12 hours after administration. Factor II (prothrombin) has a half-life of 96 hours; thus,
it can take several days to see the full antithrombotic effect of warfarin. This has an impact on dosing
regimens.

Warfarin is a drug that has the potential to interact with many other medications. These interactions
can either increase or decrease the effect of warfarin. Either way, changing the effect of a narrow
therapeutic index drug such as warfarin can cause significant harm to the patient. When a patient is
on warfarin, it is extremely important to evaluate him or her for potential drug interactions whenever
other prescription drugs, over-the-counter medications, vitamins, or alternative therapy medications are
added, discontinued, or adjusted. Due to the complexity of the warfarin-related drug interactions, it is
recommended that a pharmacist be involved in checking for interactions and recommending options
for minimizing potential interactions.

In addition to drug interactions, genetic factors, disease states, and age-related differences can affect warfarin dosing. Some patients have an enzyme-related genetic resistance to warfarin that can result in the need for 5 to 20 fold higher doses of the medication (Ronghe 2003). Patients with hepatic dysfunction do not synthesize clotting factors appropriately and require a lower dose of warfarin. Similarly, a patient with cystic fibrosis requires a lower dose of warfarin due to poor absorption of vitamin K. Newborns have decreased levels of vitamin K-dependent clotting factors and are at a greater risk of morbidity and mortality from excessive bleeding. Children do not generate as much thrombin as adults. In both of these cases, trying to achieve adult-based levels of anticoagulation in neonatal and pediatric patients can result in excessive anticoagulation.

Nursing implications

If children are prescribed warfarin in the hospital, it is likely they will have to continue it following discharge. Compliance with the medication regimen, including correct dosing, proper monitoring, and consistent follow-up, is all part of what makes warfarin therapy often challenging for families. Engage them in the process early, and reinforce the information as often as possible.

Administration and safety considerations

- ✓ Do not switch brands once a desired therapeutic effect has been achieved (Taketomo, et al., 2005).

- ✓ If you are using the injectable form of warfarin, administer it via IV only. Do not administer IM or SQ (Taketomo, et al., 2005).

- ✓ Protect tablets or injections from light (Taketomo, et al., 2005).

- ✓ Children requiring warfarin therapy will need frequent blood draws to monitor INR and other labs, especially during early use of the medication to ensure a therapeutic level. Promote child-friendly and developmentally appropriate techniques when providing comfort during blood draws or when restarting an IV. Supportive interventions include topical anesthetics, developmentally friendly containment, distraction (bubbles, storytelling, puppets, etc.), imagery, relaxation, and other techniques appropriate for the child's age and developmental level.

Teach children to eat consistently and to avoid variable intake of foods high in vitamin K (e.g., dark, leafy vegetables); they reverse the anticoagulation effects of warfarin and make titration of warfarin very difficult.

Monitoring

Prothrombin time best measures the effect on Factor VII. The assays used to measure prothrombin time can vary, so a standardized way to report the effect of warfarin on clotting factors is the international normalized ratio (INR). It is unclear how well the adult-based INR values reflect anticoagulation in pediatric patients. Pediatric patients require more monitoring and more frequent dosing adjustment than adults, making the use of this high-risk medication even riskier.

✓ Monitor INR, hemoglobin, and hematocrit levels (Taketomo, et al., 2005).

✓ Teach families about potential side effects and monitor for potential problems, including GI bleeding and systemic cholesterol microembolization (purple toes syndrome) (Taketomo, et al., 2005; McKenry and Salerno, 2003).

✓ Factors such as travel or changes in diet, environment, physical state, medications, and herbal remedies may influence the child's response to warfarin; monitor the child closely when these factors change (Taketomo, et al., 2005; Scott & Elmer, 2002).

✓ Be especially cautious of the significant effect of various drug interactions with warfarin. More than 150 medications—including over-the-counter treatments and herbal or holistic supplements—are reported to interact with warfarin (Scott & Elmer, 2002).

Parent and patient education highlights

✓ Children receiving anticoagulation therapy are more prone to bruising. This can be very challenging, especially in active children. Educate parents of this risk, and support play and activity that are developmentally appropriate with minimal risk of impact or potential injury.

✓ Use a soft toothbrush to prevent bleeding gums.

✓ Carry a medical alert identification or bracelet, if appropriate for age, to identify warfarin use (Taketomo, et al., 2005).

Case study

Teenage patient

Beth is a 16-year-old being treated with warfarin for nearly a year following heart valve replacement. Beth recently started high school and returned to her cardiologist for a routine follow-up visit as well as INR blood draw. Her exam was unremarkable, but late that night the cardiologist's office called to say that Beth's INR was extremely abnormal. Her dose was adjusted and she was scheduled to return for a repeat INR. During the follow-up blood draw, the nurse talked with Beth about any changes that had occurred that may be affecting her INR levels. Beth said she couldn't think of anything new or different. Then she told the nurse that she had recently joined the volleyball team and because she wanted to fit into a new dress for Homecoming, she had tried to eat more salads for lunch instead of going out for pizza.

1. Based on this information, what are some possible causes for the sudden change in Beth's INR?

2. What types of interventions would you suggest to Beth and her family to help Beth maintain a steady anticoagulation state in the future?

Miscellaneous anticoagulation therapies

The following classes of drugs are seldom used in pediatric patients. That alone increases their risk for error due to their relative unfamiliarity to clinicians.

Direct thrombin inhibitors

When a patient with suspected or confirmed HIT needs to continue anticoagulation, it is safe to use direct thrombin inhibitors on that patient. Like other anticoagulation therapies, most of the data on dosages and goal laboratory values is based on adult values, and the main side effect is bleeding.

Antiplatelet therapy

Although pediatric patients have platelets that are hyporeactive to thrombin, adenosine diphosphate, and thromboxane A_2, their overall bleeding time is prolonged compared to adults. Aspirin is the most common antiplatelet therapy. Slower clearance and additive effects of indomethacin or ibuprofen lysine for closure of patent ductus arteriosus are important considerations in the neonatal population. A well-known concern for pediatric patients receiving aspirin is the association with Reye's syndrome. Usually, Reye's syndrome is also associated with higher doses of aspirin (>40 mg/kg) and concomitant viral infection (Monagle, et al 2004).

Thrombolytic therapy

These agents convert endogenous plasminogen to plasmin. The lower levels of plasminogen in newborns limit the effectiveness of these agents. Although there are no head-to-head studies comparing the different agents, tPA is the drug of choice in pediatric patients. The adult absolute contraindications of stroke history, neurological disease, and hypertension should be considered as relative contraindications. There is no identified therapeutic range, and safety is often monitored by hemodynamic status. The risk of significant bleeding complications in pediatric patients has been reported to be as high as 68%, with 39% of patients requiring transfusion therapy during thrombolytic use (Monagle, et al 2004).

Chapter 6 | **Chemotherapy agents**

Learning objectives

After reading this chapter, the reader will be able to:

- Recognize why chemotherapy agents are considered pediatric high-alert medications

- Describe the chemotherapy agents most commonly used in pediatric patients

- Identify at least three ways to prevent errors when administering chemotherapeutic agents to pediatric patients

Why are chemotherapeutic agents identified as pediatric high-alert medications?

Chemotherapeutic agents are among the most potent medications given to children. Furthermore, the narrow therapeutic index and necessity of additional calculations in dosing increase the likelihood of harmful errors with chemotherapy (Rinke 2007, Kim 2006). Exact dosing and precise adherence to treatment protocols is critical to ensure that patients receive the benefits they need but without suffering undue harm. Patient deaths have resulted from unintentional overdose, inadvertent administration due to look-alike packaging or sound-alike medications, and incorrect route during administration.

Therefore, pediatric chemotherapeutic agents should be considered high-alert medications and extra safety precautions must be taken with these drugs.

Of all the classes of high-risk medications, none draws as much attention as chemotherapy. The ability of chemotherapeutic agents to cause significant toxicity is due in large part to the pathophysiology of cancer. Regardless of the cause of cancer, the result is an aberrant growth of normal human cells. Many of the traditional chemotherapeutic agents are not able to target the cause of the cancer but attack the cancerous cells instead. Although some differences between normal human cells and cancerous cells allow for a more targeted therapy, most chemotherapeutic agents are not specific enough to affect only the cancerous cells. As a result, chemotherapeutic agents result in a number of significant toxicities.

Because of the unique and unfortunate ability of chemotherapeutic agents to attack normal, healthy cells as well as cancerous cells, careful attention to correct dosing is extremely important. Although most medications have a standard adult dose or a weight-based pediatric dose, chemotherapeutic agents are generally dosed based on a patient-specific body surface area (BSA). Total drug exposure and potential toxicity are better correlated to a patient's BSA than to his or her weight (Yaffe 2005).

Therapeutic options

There are many different types of cancer with many different causes. There are also many different classes of chemotherapeutic agents. Although some chemotherapeutic agents are broad-spectrum enough to be used to treat many different types of cancer, others are specific to the treatment of a particular kind of cancer. Because so many different chemotherapeutic agents exist, each agent will not be covered. Instead, this chapter will focus on the concepts of medication safety with commonly used chemotherapeutic agents as examples.

Who is at risk?

The significant toxicities associated with chemotherapeutic agents are made even worse when a patient is not able to eliminate the toxic drugs appropriately. Therefore, young patients with immature renal function and patients with concomitant disease states that affect renal or hepatic clearance are at an increased risk of medication adverse effects. They are also at an increased risk for medication errors due to the complexities of determining the appropriate renal dose in small patients.

The use of a creatinine clearance equation to estimate renal function is a common technique in determining the renal dose of a medication. The creatinine clearance (CrCl)—generally reported in mL/min—is compared to renal dose tables in drug references that specify an adjusted dose based on the calculated value (Taketomo 2006, Robertson 2005, Micromedex). Unfortunately, pediatric patients require a different calculation that results in a "normalized" creatinine clearance that is reported in mL/min/1.73 m^2. This reflects the fact that creatinine clearance has been adjusted to the equivalent renal function for the normal or standard adult patient who is considered to have a BSA of 1.73. When the CrCl is adjusted for the patient-specific BSA, the actual—or "raw"—CrCl can be significantly lower. If this adjustment is not made, it can result in significant overdoses and serious patient harm (Liem 2003). For some drugs, such as carboplatin, there are additional calculations to help adjust the dose based on patient-specific renal function. The use of multiple calculations to determine the dose increases both the complexity of dose determination and the likelihood of significant chemotherapy overdoses.

Patients who have more aggressive types of cancer are at an increased risk for medication errors because their therapy will need to be more aggressive. Multiple agents are often used to attack the cancer by several different mechanisms. Each chemotherapeutic agent that is added to a patient's regimen adds additional risks. Some of these risks are obvious, such as additional side effects and drug interactions when different agents are combined. But multiple medications also pose subtler risks, such as additional opportunities for a prescribing, dispensing, or administration errors.

Carboplatin case

A 6-year-old girl with one kidney is to receive carboplatin as part of her therapy for Wilms tumor. In the absence of a renal scan, the Glomerular Filtration Rate (GFR) is estimated by the pediatric CrCl calculation (Schwartz Formula) to be 83 mL/min/1.73 (Taketomo 2006). This value is plugged into a dosing calculation (modified Calvert formula) that yielded a dose of 545 mg of carboplatin (Liem 2003). This dose looked high to the nurse caring for the little girl, so she sought clarification from the ordering physician and the pharmacy before administering the dose. The nurse was assured by the physician and pharmacy that the creatinine clearance was calculated appropriately. The nurse continued to feel unsettled about the confusing order and sought additional clarification. Upon closer look by another practitioner, the modified Calvert formula required the GFR estimate to be in units of mL/min (raw CrCl), NOT mL/min/1.73 m^2 (normalized CrCl) as calculated by the Schwartz Formula. When 83 mL/min/1.73 m^2 is divided by 1.73 and multiplied by the patient's BSA of 0.85 m^2, the patient-specific CrCl of 41 mL/min is the result. Thus, the GFR estimate that was included in the equation was more than two times the estimate that should have been used. The actual dose should have been only 300 mg. Thanks to the nurse's attention to detail, the patient who already had kidney damage, was spared an 80% overdose of a toxic chemotherapeutic agent that is renally eliminated from the body.

1. Name two things that went wrong during the medication use process for this chemotherapeutic agent.

2. What did the nurse do correctly?

3. What steps can you implement in your hospital to avoid a similar near-miss with carboplatin?

More aggressive therapy may lead to such significant organ toxicities that they have lifetime maximum dosing limits. The toxicity of aggressive chemotherapy often requires the administration of protective agents to limit toxicity. Even if the protective agents have minimal side-effect or drug interaction potential, the addition of extra medications to a patient's profile makes the patient's profile more complex to review and may cause the physician to overlook a more serious concern.

Lastly, treating aggressive cancer does not involve only medications; it may also involve radiation therapy. Radiation has its own side-effect profiles that may overlap with the toxicities from certain chemotherapeutic medications. This can require lower doses of chemotherapy, which is easy to overlook when focusing on only drug–drug interactions.

Because of the high risk associated with chemotherapy, much of the treatment is based on study protocols that carefully spell out each chemotherapeutic regimen. For pediatric oncology, these official study protocols are consolidated into one place, the Children's Oncology Group (*www.childrensoncologygroup.org*). This adds an element of safety in that the regimens are being studied closely, and the dosing directions and timing of administration are readily available in what is called a *road map*.

Patients who are not able to be treated according to protocol are at an increased risk of medication errors. Whenever a patient is treated off-protocol or off-study, extra attention should be taken to verify the chemotherapy dosing and timing of administration. As much as possible, use a process that reflects a protocol approach to off-protocol chemotherapy treatments. Even though a formalized road map may not be available, the attending oncologist's plan for therapy should be similarly written out so that all practitioners know what drugs the patient is to receive at what time in a course of therapy that may last for months.

Due to the complex regimens and detailed protocols for chemotherapeutic agents, preprinted order sheets can be used to enhance safety and reduce errors. Handwritten orders increase the risk for errors due to potential issues with illegibility and because they must be written separately for each patient. Furthermore, handwritten orders may not be seen and checked by another practitioner, whereas preprinted orders are generally reviewed and validated by several clinicians before being approved, thus adding the extra safety of multiple reviewers.

Patients who are not treated by an active, multidisciplinary team also may be at risk for increased medication errors. The complexities of treating cancer are best managed when experts from the medical, nursing, pharmacy, and other support services are involved in a patient's care. The more specialists involved, the more attention to detail for that particular specialty. For example, a physician, a nurse, and a pharmacist may check the same set of orders, yet find different mistakes and opportunities for clarifying them. If possible, a system that allows for two physicians, two nurses, and two pharmacists to review every order is ideal. In this model, two physicians review the orders initially before sending them to pharmacy. Two independent pharmacists check the order for appropriateness. In addition to the order entry pharmacist who serves as the first check, the second pharmacist could be a clinical specialist, the pharmacist checking the final product before dispensing, or another pharmacist unrelated to the preparation of the chemotherapy. Finally, the administering nurse should have a fellow nurse double-check the chemotherapy product against the order before administering the medication. All of these double-checks take time, and squeezing this extra time into a busy pediatric hematology–oncology service can be difficult. However, the added safety benefit of multiple clinician checks can be well worth the time.

Patients are also at an increased risk of medication errors when the time frame allotted to the ordering, dispensing, and administration processes is inadequate. When the steps in these processes are rushed, there is an opportunity for error: a trailing zero on an order that leads to a tenfold overdose, selecting vincristine instead of vinblastine upon order entry, or hanging the wrong bag on the wrong patient. All of these errors can lead to significant patient harm when clinicians are rushed to perform their critical jobs in a hasty manner.

Pediatric considerations

Epidemiology

Children are less likely to develop cancer than adults. Pediatric patients who develop cancer are more likely to recover and have a greater chance of survival than adults who develop cancer (Rowland 2005). It is difficult to determine whether children who develop and are treated for cancer are at greater risk for being diagnosed with another cancer later in life. When this does occur, there is still the question of whether the second cancer is related to the original one, as a result of chemotherapy regimens used in treating the first cancer, or simply a coincidence.

Physiology

Much of cancer pathophysiology has to do with disruption of the cell replication process. These processes can change in respect to age. Typically, pediatric patients have a higher turnover of cells and increased cell replication. This may set patients up for a cancer, or it may mask the effects of cancerous cells that might otherwise lead to diagnosis of cancer in adults. The rapid turnover of cells may also contribute to a pediatric patient's improved response to treatment compared to adults.

Pharmacokinetics

Some chemotherapy agents are given intramuscularly. In infants and younger children, intramuscular (IM) medications are absorbed inconsistently. Therefore, it is best to avoid the use of this route of administration if possible. When an IM injection is needed in an infant or young child, the volume per injection site should be reduced to 1 mL per site for young children and 0.5 mL per site for infants. Depending on the drug, the differences in pediatric pharmacokinetics can either increase or decrease the elimination. For the most part, hepatic metabolism is increased in pediatric patients, and renal excretion is decreased in neonates, infants, and young children. This may affect dosing of certain chemotherapeutic agents such as methotrexate, which require clearance of drug levels to a lower limit before redosing can occur.

Drug formulations

Most dosage forms—particularly oral dosage forms—are not made for pediatric patients. Because pediatric patients are often unable to swallow pills, liquid forms of oral chemotherapeutic agents are often extemporaneously prepared by pharmacies. Any preparation that involves compounding of a manufactured dosage form has an added risk of drug error.

Even when a pediatric patient can swallow a tablet, the tablet may need to be cut or split to an appropriate dosage form. This adds the risk that the patient may get too little or too much of the medication. It can also lead to dosing confusion if a particular regimen requires a patient to alternate between whole and half tablets during the course of a week. This is not an uncommon practice in dosing oral chemotherapy agents in children, but one that does represent an opportunity for increased safety through standardized doses (Taylor 2006).

Drug indications and medical management

The types of cancer that affect pediatric patients are different from those that affect adults. Solid and liquid tumors can affect both age groups. However, the incidences of the types of solid and liquid tumors are very different. For example, acute lymphocytic leukemia is more common in children, whereas acute myelogenous leukemia is more common in adults. The common sites for pediatric solid tumors are the brain and the kidney. In adults, however, lung, breast, colon, and prostate are more common forms of cancer.

The difference in the types of cancer that affect pediatric patients leads to a very different approach to chemotherapy. The drugs, doses, and durations of therapy that are used in treating pediatric cancer are very different from those used in treating adult cancer. For this reason, a separate group of protocols exists for treating pediatric patients. Occasionally, there is crossover of an adult protocol used in a pediatric patient. However, this generally occurs in an older child or adolescent when a patient has relapsed after treatment with several pediatric protocols.

Compliance

There are many issues with compliance when it comes to treating pediatric oncology patients. To start with, most medications are designed for adults. This makes administration of oral tablets difficult for patients who cannot swallow tablets or who require very small doses.

Compliance is made even more difficult for patients who are nauseated or vomiting. These patients can become very particular about the medications they take based on prior experiences. For example, some patients will refuse all liquid medications if they associate previous episodes of nausea and vomiting with liquid medications. These kinds of compliance issues affect not only the chemotherapy agents but also any oral medication that a patient may take, such as ondansetron orally disintegrating tablets.

The administration of intravenous products is easier from a preparation standpoint, although obtaining adequate, long-term line access for chemotherapy regimens can be difficult. This is even harder in younger patients, who do not comprehend the need for the line and try to pull it out.

Compliance issues also can extend beyond taking medications. Some chemotherapeutic regimens have significant toxicities that require careful nonpharmacologic plans to limit toxicity. For example, the chemotherapy drug thiotepa is excreted through the skin and can cause significant skin burns. Therefore, therapy with thiotepa requires multiple showers per day to protect the skin from the drug. Some pediatric patients have a hard time tolerating showers and baths, making this necessary plan difficult to carry out for the patient and his or her caregiver.

Drug-specific information

Busulfan: Dosing requires pharmacokinetic equations, which can increase the risk of dosing errors.

Cisplatin/carboplatin: Avoid look-alike/sound-alike issues.

Cyclophosphamide: Avoid the abbreviations CTX, CPM, and CYT; requires Mesna as a renal protectant.

Cytarabine: Avoid the abbreviation ARA-C.

Dactinomycin: Do not confuse with the antibiotic daptomycin.

Daunorubicin/doxorubicin: Avoid look-alike/sound-alike issues.

Etoposide/teniposide: Avoid look-alike/sound-alike issues.

Ifosfamide: Requires Mesna as a renal protectant.

L-asparaginase/pegaspargase/erwinia l-asparaginase: All three of these agents can be easy to confuse. The first is the original *E. coli*-derived enzyme. Pegaspargase is the pegylated form of *E. coli* l-asparaginase designed to reduce side effects. Erwinia l-asparaginase is from a different origin for patients with hypersensitivity to *E. coli* l-asparaginase products; it is only available as an investigational agent.

Methotrexate: Careful attention must be paid to levels after administration; if levels are not coming down appropriately, use leucovorin to help reduce the toxic effects.

Topotecan/irinotecan: Avoid look-alike/sound-alike issues.

Vinblastine/vincristine/vinorelbine: Avoid look-alike/sound-alike issues.

5-fluorouracil: Avoid the abbreviation 5-FU.

6-mercaptopurine: Avoid the abbreviation 6-MP; avoid look-alike/sound-alike issue with 6-thioguanine.

6-thioguanine: Avoid the abbreviation 6-TG; avoid look-alike/sound-alike issue with 6-mercaptopurine.

Nursing implications

Chemotherapy administration protocols require a coordinated, well-educated, multidisciplinary approach involving oncologists, pharmacists, nurses, patients and their families, and when available, certified child life specialists. Use the "keep kids safe" section in chapter 4 for advice on tips and strategies for all high-alert medications.

Administration and safety considerations for chemotherapy

Safe chemotherapy administration begins long before the medication is prepared and administered. Some of the key safety considerations include:

✓ Ensure that consent for the treatment protocol has been signed and is in the patient's chart prior to the start of any chemotherapy regimen.

✓ Accept chemotherapy orders from certified prescribers only (Kline et al. 2004).

✓ No verbal orders or telephone orders should be accepted for chemotherapy agents, except to discontinue or hold a medication (Kline et al. 2004).

✓ Chemotherapy-certified nurses, nurses who have received additional training (didactic and clinical demonstration) in the use of chemotherapeutic agents, or oncology physicians should be the only people administering chemotherapeutic agents (Kline et al. 2004).

✓ Prior to administering a chemotherapy medication, the nurse must do the following (Kline, et al., 2004):

 – Ensure that he or she is treating the correct patient, by using two different identifiers

 – Verify allergy status

 – Verify premedication orders

 – Verify that a complete and accurate chemotherapy order, including physician signature, has been issued

 – Recalculate the patient's BSA

 – Recalculate the drug dosage

 – Compare the dose on the drug label to the dose on the original order

    – Verify that the proper double-checks were completed by the pharmacy department and that signatures or initials are complete according to institutional policy

    – Calculate the infusion rate

    – Confirm the correct route

✓ The "Right" sequence and timing of drugs is another "Right" in safe chemotherapy administration (Kline et al. 2004).

✓ Follow hospital or institution-specific guidelines for safe chemotherapy ordering, dispensing, handling, administration, and disposal, as well as for the handling and disposal of patient waste. (Kline et al. 2004).

✓ Independent double-checks of the order, prepared chemotherapy solution, and rate and route of administration are crucial.

✓ If there is ever a question about a chemotherapeutic order or prepared chemotherapy solution, *stop the line,* and review the process with everyone involved.

✓ Have the chemotherapy protocol at the patient's bedside or wherever chemotherapy is being administered.

✓ When administering chemotherapy IV, flush the line well before and after medication administration using the prescribed flush volume and solution. Ensure that the line has been completely cleared of the medication and that the patient has received the entire dose of the chemotherapeutic agent (Kline et al. 2004).

Stop the line is a safety term first coined by the Toyota Production System. In short, it means any member of the team can stop the production line—or in healthcare terms, stop whatever process, procedure, or intervention is taking place—and the team will attend to the safety issue. The person that stopped the line is not punished for stopping "production" but rather is supported for addressing safety issues on the spot.

Monitoring

✓ Acquire a CBC with differential, and other labs as ordered or as required according to the treatment protocol (Kline et al. 2004).

✓ Monitor and document the effectiveness of the chemotherapy treatment regimen, including any side effects (Kline et al. 2004).

✓ Know the potential complications or side effects associated with the class of chemotherapy agent in use. Have the necessary equipment available to respond to expected or unexpected responses to the treatment. (Kline et al. 2004).

Patient and family education highlights

✓ Teach the patient and his or her family about the treatment plan using age-appropriate and developmentally appropriate language and methods. Include the names of medications, the planned and expected schedules for treatments, and possible side effects (Kline et al. 2004).

✓ Remind the patient and family about side effects that may be immediate and others that could occur over time, maybe even over days or weeks (Kline et al. 2004).

✓ Instruct the patient and family how to handle chemotherapy waste, including waste contained in body fluids. Instruct the family of any special precautions that may be required when disposing of diapers, changing linens, and so on (Kline et al. 2004).

Case study

Underdosing

A patient with a body surface area of 1 m² was ordered to receive PEG L-asparaginase 2,500 units IM once. However, the pharmacy misinterpreted the drug name and filled the order with non-pegylated L-asparaginase 2,500 units. The fact that the usual dosing of L-asparaginase is 10,000 units/m² per dose was not caught when the order was double-checked before dispensing.

1. What two "Rights" were violated in this pharmacist error?

2. What could nurses have done to prevent this error from reaching the patient?

Case study

Danger of waste

A new pediatric hematology-oncology nurse is anxiously waiting for her patient's chemotherapy to arrive from pharmacy so she can take him to radiology for a scheduled lumbar puncture and intrathecal (IT) medication administration. When the pharmacy tech finally shows up with her patient's chemo, she grabs everything for her patient and rushes off to radiology. She brings the vincristine, cytarabine, and a few other meds into the procedure room, figuring the few extra syringes will not clutter things up too much. During the procedure, the distracted physician grabbed the vincristine syringe instead of the cytarabine syringe and administered it intrathecally. The patient reacted poorly after the procedure and was transferred to the PICU where he died a few days later. Vincristine is a vesicant that is fatal when given by the intrathecal route. This error is a current focus of the World Health Organization, The Joint Commission, and the ISMP (ISMP Medication Safety Alert. December 2005)

1. What series of events played a role in this fatal mistake?

2. What is in place in your institution to keep high-alert medication errors such as this from occurring?

Chapter 7 | **Concentrated electrolytes**

Learning objectives

After reading this chapter, the reader will be able to:

- Recognize why concentrated electrolytes are considered pediatric high-alert medications

- Describe the concentrated electrolytes most commonly used in pediatric patients

- Identify at least three ways to prevent errors when administering concentrated electrolytes to pediatric patients

Why are concentrated electrolytes identified as pediatric high-alert medications?

On the surface, electrolytes are an unlikely candidate for high-risk medications because they simply supplement substances that are naturally present in our bodies. However, electrolytes are among the most lethal medications that are administered in a hospital setting. The risk electrolytes pose is overlooked partly because they are often not considered medications; however, the U.S. Food and Drug Administration's definition of a drug in the Federal Food, Drug, and Cosmetic Act is any substance intended to affect the structure or function of the body. Clearly this applies to electrolytes.

Like other high-alert medications, errors have been the result of incorrect dosing, look-alike packaging, erroneous dispensing, and infusion mistakes.

Hospitalized and sick children often require electrolyte therapies to maintain fluid and electrolyte homeostasis, a crucial part of their ongoing treatment. Errors associated with concentrated electrolytes in children can be devastating. Overdoses or underdoses that may seem insignificant can actually cause significant morbidity and mortality.

The danger of electrolytes is often underestimated, evident by the fact that they were historically kept in high concentrations throughout hospitals. Although pharmacies were required to store and prepare other hazardous medications, concentrated electrolytes such as 2 mEq/mL potassium chloride were readily available on nursing units. Even small amounts of potassium chloride can be fatal when administered undiluted. Fortunately, The Joint Commission put an end to this practice and brought the danger of electrolytes to the forefront with National Patient Safety Goal 3A, calling for removal of concentrated electrolytes from units (The Joint Commission 2003).

Therapeutic options

All of the naturally occurring electrolytes in the body are available commercially. Because electrolytes are ionic molecules, they only exist outside the body in a salt form. For example, it is not possible to give a dose of sodium alone. To give a dose of sodium to a patient, sodium chloride, sodium acetate, or sodium phosphate must be used. The fact that electrolytes are only available as pairs is both helpful and complicating. If a patient needs replacement of sodium and chloride, we can accomplish both with one drug. However, if we wanted to increase the chloride for a patient who also had a high serum sodium level, sodium chloride would not be an option. Fortunately, the commercially available electrolytes come in a variety of combinations that allow us to fine-tune a patient's serum electrolyte status (see Figure 7.1).

Because two electrolytes are present in each drug combination, care must be taken when communicating about electrolytes in a clinical context. For example, if a physician gives a verbal order for 20 mEq of sodium IV over two hours, the order is incomplete and could lead to an error. The physician must specify if the sodium will be given as sodium chloride or sodium acetate.

| Figure 7.1 | Commercially available intravenous electrolyte combinations |

| Sodium chloride |
| Sodium acetate |
| Sodium bicarbonate |
| Sodium phosphate |
| Potassium chloride |
| Potassium acetate |
| Potassium phosphate |
| Calcium chloride |
| Calcium gluconate |
| Magnesium sulfate |
| Magnesium chloride |

Source: Lexi-Comp 2006.

The order of how the electrolyte combinations are named reflects their chemical structure with the *cation* (positively charged ion) listed first (e.g., sodium chloride = Na^+ Cl^-). This usually reflects the clinical importance of the electrolytes as well. Of the five most commonly used electrolytes, four are positive ions (sodium, potassium, calcium, and magnesium). Phosphorous is the most commonly used *anion* (negatively charged ion). This can sometimes lead to confusion because the generic names for all phosphorous supplements start with the name of another electrolyte. To account for this, some drug reference books will list the various dosage forms under the heading "Phosphate Supplements" rather than by the individual chemical names (Lexi-Comp 2006).

The naming issues of electrolytes extend beyond the drug name to the units used to describe the dose. Because the electrolytes exist as the salt form of ionic molecules, the most common units used to describe the amount of the electrolytes are milliequivalents (mEq). A milliequivalent is a way to relate the weight of an electrolyte substance to its molecular weight. The benefit of using milliequivalents is that the term refers to the individual strength of each electrolyte in the salt form. For example, 10 mEq of sodium chloride refers to 10 mEq of sodium and 10 mEq of chloride. In this way, the dose of the elemental form of the sodium is clear.

Sometimes the strengths of electrolytes are converted to a milligram amount. Although milligram is a more familiar term to clinicians when dosing drugs, the use of milligrams when dosing electrolytes can be confusing because they can refer to the entire salt combination or to just one of the elements. For example, intravenous calcium gluconate is available as a 100 mg/mL concentration. This reflects the amount of the calcium and gluconate in one mL, or the amount of the entire salt form. Of that 100 mg/mL, only 9 mg/mL is actual elemental calcium. It is important to keep in mind that from a physiologic perspective, the elemental amount of electrolytes is what counts. Although dosing algorithms may reflect either the salt form or the elemental form of calcium, it is essential to know on which form the dose is based. In the case of calcium gluconate, if a 50 mg/kg dose based on the salt form is filled as 50 mg/kg based on the elemental form, a greater than tenfold overdose could result.

In addition to naming considerations, there are dosing considerations when using various salt forms of a given electrolyte. For example, calcium chloride is also available as a 100 mg/mL salt concentration. However, the amount of elemental calcium in the calcium chloride salt is 27.2 mg/mL—three times the amount of elemental calcium per milliliter. With so much potential for error in dosing intravenous electrolytes with different salts, it is wise to select one consistent method for dosing electrolytes throughout an institution.

Although ordering units for electrolytes are not specifically mentioned, the American Academy of Pediatrics Policy Statement on prevention of pediatric inpatient medication errors does recommend the standardization of measurements (AAP 2003). It would seem reasonable that such standardization would also apply to measuring medications. Milligrams of salt, elemental milligrams, or milliequivalents can all be safely used, as long as only one of the three is consistently used to order, dispense, and administer electrolytes. Milliequivalents would seem to be the safest choice because it refers to the elemental strength of the individual electrolytes and has the least potential for confusion between salt forms. For example, even in a system that standardizes doses to elemental magnesium, there is still the potential for a significant overdose if a given practitioner orders an electrolyte based on the milligrams of the salt form without specifying that in the order. The pharmacist and nurse who are used to dealing with doses in elemental milligrams may interpret the order as being in elemental milligrams. While the pharmacist or nurse may catch such an error by the high dose, this can often be overlooked in a pediatric environment. The reason for this is the wide range of pediatric weights leading to a wide range of final doses. What may look like a "normal" dose of 2 grams of IV calcium gluconate would be a significant overdose for a 5 kg patient. This underscores the importance of weight-based dosing in pediatrics. Although milliequivalents seems like the best choice since there is no opportunity for salt/elemental confusion, there are no formal recommendations or studies that confirm that using milliequivalents is the safest dosing unit to use. Indeed, changing from one dosing method to another may create additional error within a given hospital system, so each hospital should evaluate the safest dosing method for its patient population.

Who is at risk?

The greatest risk of errors with electrolytes occurs in patients who are receiving intravenous supplementation. The toxic and potentially life-threatening effects of electrolyte overdoses occur when larger than physiologic amounts of electrolytes are present at target end organs such as the brain and the heart. Intravenous administration allows for direct, concentrated amounts of electrolytes to be delivered rapidly to the heart and subsequently to the brain. Even with dilution in the bloodstream, significant clinical overdoses are possible with a simple tenfold dosing error. However, when overdoses are administered enterally, there is less risk of patient harm. There are limits to the amount of electrolytes that can be absorbed at one time. Excess amounts of acutely administered electrolytes are simply lost through the gastrointestinal tract or filtered by the kidneys. Chronic overload of electrolytes is still possible with oral administration, but this develops slowly and usually with a less severe clinical presentation.

Patients who have concomitant disease states are at a greater risk for chronic electrolyte overload. For example, patients with kidney dysfunction are more likely to have chronic accumulations of potassium and phosphorous, even with normal nutritional intake. Concomitant disease states also put patients at a greater risk for increases or decreases in electrolytes due to drug–drug interactions. Diuretics can significantly increase or decrease the serum concentrations of electrolytes. Patients with disease states or medications that result in electrolyte wasting are at an increased risk for medication errors due to the large amount of parenteral supplementation required to maintain physiologic electrolyte concentrations. They are also at risk for the effects of inadequate supplementation if consistent, careful attention is not paid to their electrolyte status.

When patients are receiving all of their nutrition parenterally, it may seem that they would be at less risk of electrolyte disorders due to the simplicity of bypassing the gastrointestinal tract for all electrolyte supplementation. However, this actually increases their risk. In addition to the risks associated with intravenous electrolytes discussed earlier, there is more opportunity for error due to the complex processes associated with total parenteral nutrition (TPN) preparation. Overdoses or underdoses are possible, depending on the type of error in preparation. Furthermore, there is less ability to titrate doses of individual electrolytes when one intravenous solution includes all of a patient's electrolytes. Sometimes, TPNs will need to be held or stopped for a period of time due to one elevated lab result. This in turn affects all of the micronutrients and macronutrients in that day's TPN bag.

Pediatric considerations

Epidemiology

Due to the increased fluid and electrolyte requirements, unique aspects of feeding, and immature organ systems in children, the use of electrolytes in the pediatric population is more complex than in adults. Therefore, there is a greater need to carefully monitor and frequently replace electrolytes in children.

Physiology

Fluid and electrolyte needs are based on metabolic rate, not simply body weight. The metabolic rate per kg of bodyweight decreases with increasing age. Therefore, children need more fluid and electrolytes per kg of bodyweight compared to adults but less fluid and electrolytes per kg of bodyweight than neonates and infants (Roberts 2001).

Because fluid needs are increased for smaller patients, a greater percentage of fluid-based weight loss is required for diagnosis of dehydration in children than in adults. For example, moderate dehydration in a pediatric patient is defined as a 10% loss of body weight, whereas it is only 5% in an adult (Roberts 2001).

Pharmacokinetics

Since the electrolytes distribute, at least in part, to the fluid compartments of the body, the changes in fluid status in growing children will also affect the distribution of electrolytes. This is especially true for sodium, which is an extra cellular electrolyte (i.e., an electrolyte that is found predominantly in extra cellular fluid.)

The kidney plays a key role in regulating the body's stores of electrolytes. In the developing infant, there are immaturities in glomerular filtration and in the ability to concentrate the urine. This does not necessarily change the approach to dosing neonates and infants with electrolytes, but it should be kept in mind when interpreting a patient's lab results.

Drug formulations

Concentrated formulations make pediatric dosing easier but increase risks for fatal overdoses. Although it might be convenient to store electrolytes on the unit for easy replacement, the deadly risks of a small patient receiving an undiluted bolus is too great. If dilute forms of commonly administered electrolytes are desired to be kept on a busy unit, there will be stability and storage issues to keep in mind. Because each of the major electrolytes comes in various salt forms, there could also be safety issues with storing multiple salt forms on a given unit. For example, a nurse may inadvertently grab calcium chloride when calcium gluconate was the intended drug. If the calcium chloride is then inadvertently administered via a peripheral line, the patient could experience an adverse drug event. Except for emergency medications, it is safer to provide routine electrolyte replacement doses from the pharmacy.

Drug indications

The drug indications are the same in children as in adults: maintenance of physiologic electrolyte concentrations. Following laboratory values does not always tell the whole story, especially for intracellular electrolytes such as potassium where the majority of the body's stores are not available to be measured in the bloodstream. Looking for signs and symptoms of electrolyte abnormalities can differ in children. For example, dehydration may be best observed by a sunken fontanel and tachycardia rather than looking at blood urea nitrogen:serum creatinine ratios (Robertson 2005).

Medical management

Because pediatric patients have a greater percentage of total body water, infants and young children need a greater volume per kg rescue bolus. Despite the different volume needs and varying levels of pharmacokinetic maturity, the same sodium concentrations found in maintenance fluid are appropriate for infants and children (Roberts 2001).

Compliance

This is a legitimate concern with oral electrolyte supplementation. The saltiness of the oral dosage forms is difficult for many patients to tolerate. There is more than one way to improve the palatability of the oral formulations, and a plan should be tailored to each patient's specific preferences. Options for improving palatability include mixing the oral supplementation with other liquids such as juice or formula, numbing or blocking the taste buds with a popsicle or peanut butter before administering the supplement, and following the supplement with a favorite food to help remove the aftertaste.

Even with the various masking techniques, some patients still do not tolerate oral supplements and may have trouble keeping them down. When this occurs, intravenous supplementation or other techniques may be necessary. For example, when mild sodium replacement is needed but oral formulations are not tolerated, it is sometimes recommended that pediatric patients simply increase their intake of salty foods. This decision, however, should be made with consideration of the patient's overall nutritional needs and restrictions.

Drug-specific information

Sodium (Na⁺)

Importance: Water follows sodium in the body, so of all the electrolytes, sodium has the greatest effect on fluid shifts and balances in the body. It is also important in neuromuscular function, water regulation in the kidney, and maintenance of acid-base balance, potassium, and chloride levels (Elgart 2004).

Special considerations: Rapid elevation or lowering of sodium levels can lead to severe neurological consequences such as seizures or brain herniation as water is either pulled out of or pushed into the brain from the bloodstream to equilibrate the sodium–water balance.

It is necessary to determine the appropriate treatment by identifying the patient's hydration status along with sodium status. Concentrated sodium chloride (above a physiological concentration of 0.9% sodium chloride) should be used with caution and should never be stored outside the pharmacy or with other sodium chloride bags that look similar.

Normal saline (0.9% sodium chloride; 154 mEq/mL) should be used for initial fluid resuscitation and one-half normal saline (0.45% sodium chloride; 77 mEq/mL) should be used for replacing sodium chloride deficits. One-quarter normal saline can be a little confusing. Technically, it is 0.225% sodium chloride (38.5 mEq/mL). However, for simplicity, it is manufactured and generally prepared as 0.2% sodium chloride (34.2 mEq/mL). The difference of 4.3 mEq is not clinically significant, and either 0.225% or 0.2% sodium chloride can be used to provide maintenance fluid when combined with dextrose 5% or 10% (Roberts 2001).

Potassium (K⁺)

Importance: Potassium's most important role is in regulating muscular activity, including the cardiac muscle. It is also involved in maintaining cellular osmolarity equilibrium, enzyme activation, and acid-base balance (Elgart 2004).

Special considerations: Hyperkalemia can lead to minor ECG changes at serum levels of 5.5–6 mEq/L and fatal aystole at levels of >8 mEq/L (Elgart 2004). Because of this, intravenous administration must be done with care. Drug references list the maximum safe infusion rates for patients with and without continuous EKG monitoring. They also list the maximum safe concentrations for administration in peripheral or central lines. Many hospitals have institution-specific policies that may be more conservative or liberal than the drug references

Acidosis, medications, and trauma can all increase potassium levels. Heel sticks in neonates can lead to falsely elevated potassium levels due to excess potassium release from the local trauma (Elgart 2004).

Signs and symptoms of hypokalemia may not be recognized until blood levels reach 3 mEq/L. Replacement of potassium must be estimated due to the majority of the body's supplies being in the cells. Usually, 40 mEq/L of potassium will increase the plasma concentration by 1 mEq/mL (Elgart 2004).

Magnesium (Mg⁺⁺)

Importance: Magnesium has many important functions regarding intracellular metabolism, enzyme activation, sodium and potassium transport, and intracellular calcium regulation (Elgart 2004).

Special considerations: Toxicity ranges from minor weakness and flushing at levels >4 mg/dL to complete heart block, paralysis, cardiac arrest, and respiratory arrest at levels >10 mg/dL (Elgart 2004).

Dosing can be expressed in terms of mg of salt, mg of magnesium, or mEq. Orders should be kept consistent within a hospital system. Rapid administration of replacement doses may result in acute toxicity and ineffective replacement. Instead, replacement doses should be given over four to six hours.

Calcium (Ca⁺⁺)

Importance: Calcium's most noticeable role is in bone formation and development, but it is also important in neuromuscular and enzyme activity as well as in coagulation of the blood (Elgart 2004).

Special considerations: Blood levels may not reflect total body stores. Blood levels also can be measured in two ways: as bound to protein or in its ionized form. The ionized form is the form that the body can actually use and is a more accurate reflection of calcium available in the blood stream, because low protein levels can lead to a lower than actual serum calcium level.

Calcium can bind to phosphorous and cause problems either inside intravenous tubing or inside the patient. Care should be taken when administering calcium with other medications through the same infusion site. Keep in mind that the calcium and phosphorous may be present in IV fluids and TPN as well.

Calcium comes in many salt forms. The amount of actual calcium administered to the patient can vary significantly depending on the salt forms used. To avoid confusion and complications in dosing, choose dosing units of mEq or mg of elemental calcium.

To enhance absorption and eliminate side effects, slow infusion over four to six hours is recommended. Sometimes when calcium is used for its positive inotropic effects, it is administered as a continuous infusion. When this is done, care must be taken in calculating the hourly rate to avoid providing calcium dosing above appropriate daily limits. In addition, if patients are receiving calcium from several sources (TPN, continuous infusion, intermittent supplementation in enteral feeds), monitoring ionized calcium levels is appropriate to ensure that the patient is not receiving toxic amounts of calcium.

Phosphorus

Importance: Phosphorus is an important source of cellular energy for the body. It also helps regulate calcium and acid-base balance and has a role in carbohydrate and lipid metabolism (Elgart 2004).

Special considerations: Dosing of phosphorous can be confusing because it is often reported in units of mMol/L rather than mEq/L. This is because it does not exist as an electrolyte by itself but rather in combination with four oxygen molecules. It can also be expressed in terms of mg. To further add to the confusion, the potassium content of potassium phosphate is reported in terms of mEq/L.

When patients are malnourished, adequate replacement of phosphate is essential before nutrition to avoid refeeding syndrome (Kraft 2005). Adequate phosphorous supplementation is also essential in patients who are being extubated. The energy provided by phosphorous during the respiration process is important as patients move from being ventilated to maintaining their breathing on their own.

Nursing implications

As mentioned at the beginning of this chapter, The Joint Commission, IHI and ISMP recommend that all concentrated electrolytes are removed from floor stock areas. The first concentrated electrolyte most people think of removing is potassium chloride. It is, without a doubt, extremely dangerous and potentially lethal. However, all concentrated electrolytes have the potential to produce devastating outcomes if the dose is prepared or administered incorrectly. In fact, many pediatric pharmacy departments treat the most dangerous concentrated electrolytes (such as hypertonic >0.9% sodium chloride and potassium chloride) like a controlled substance and keep these solutions in locked cabinets to minimize the chance of unintended administration. Nurses should never be in a position of adding concentrated electrolytes to other solutions or the mixing of intravenous fluids. The rare exception might include emergency departments, transport teams, and during extreme ICU emergency situations. Even in these instances, institutions should develop a plan for how these high-alert medications will be stored, prescribed, prepared and administered and consider all possible alternatives and processes for keeping concentrated electrolytes out of floor stock and in the pharmacy (IHI).

Administration and safety considerations

Some of the key safety considerations with electrolytes include:

✓ Remove concentrated electrolytes from all floor stock areas (IHI).

✓ Determine the cause of the electrolyte imbalance, and treat it with electrolyte correction as well as by addressing the underlying causes for the imbalance.

✓ Institutions and nursing units should agree on standard intravenous electrolyte solutions, significantly decreasing the number of steps (and potential for error) in pharmacy IVF preparation (IHI).

✓ Require the pharmacy to review all orders (IHI).

✓ Administer electrolyte replacement infusions via a central line whenever possible.

✓ Take caution when piggybacking electrolyte infusions into a maintenance fluid that already contains electrolytes, especially if infusing via a peripheral IV line. Be cognizant that piggybacking may dramatically change the fluid osmolality (Taketomo, et al. 2005).

Monitoring

✓ Due to the potential for sudden changes in respiratory and cardiac stability, continuous ECG and pulse oximetry should be used during corrective electrolyte infusions (McKenry & Salerno 2003).

✓ If one electrolyte laboratory result is drastically different from a previous result, discuss with the physician and consider redrawing before attempting to correct using concentrated electrolyte fluids. (McKenry and Salerno (2003).

✓ Monitor glucose, intake and output, weight, and renal function (Taketomo, et al. 2005).

✓ Monitor the patient's peripheral IV sites closely. Concentrated electrolyte infiltrates can result in potential tissue necrosis and extravasation (Taketomo, et al. 2005).

Note: What is the diference between ionized and serum calcium?

Ionized calcium is free-flowing and readily available because it is not attached to proteins. Serum calcium is the total calcium, including calcium that is bound to protein and not so easily available. Because serum calcium levels are affected by albumin levels, calcium levels are often best assessed by monitoring ionized calcium levels.

Patient and family education highlights

✓ Educate the child and family about how to recognize signs and symptoms of hypo- and hyper- states as they relate to the electrolyte imbalance being treated

✓ Discuss ways in which electrolyte imbalances can be addressed by diet, when appropriate

Sodium:

✓ Hypertonic sodium chloride (>0.9%) should be stored in a secure location, separate from other sodium chloride or diluent solutions, to avoid inadvertent misuse (IHI)

✓ Hypertonic saline less than 0.2% should never be infused alone

Potassium:

✓ Place the patient on a continuous cardiac monitor during intermittent potassium replacement infusions (Taketomo, C., et al. 2005)

✓ IV potassium chloride should be stored in a secure location (IHI)

✓ IV potassium chloride must always be diluted (Taketomo, C., et al. 2005; McKenry and Salerno 2003)

✓ Potassium chloride should *never* be given IVP (Taketomo, C., et al. 2005)

✓ Do not crush or chew tablets (Taketomo, C., et al. 2005)

✓ Administer tablets with food or a large glass of water to minimize GI upset (Taketomo, et al., 2005)

Calcium:

✓ *Never* administer IM or SQ. Calcium can cause severe tissue necrosis (Taketomo, C., et al. 2005).

✓ Infuse calcium using a central line, whenever possible. Because of the potential risk for tissue necrosis or extravasation, administer calcium cautiously in small hand, foot, or scalp veins. (Taketomo, C., et al. 2005).

✓ Some units store two types of calcium solutions, especially in emergency carts. Be extremely cautious if both calcium chloride and calcium gluconate are available. Calcium chloride is extremely irritating if administered into a peripheral intravenous line (PIV) and should never be given IM (ISMP 1997).

Magnesium:

✓ Monitor respiratory status closely for signs of decreased respiratory drive or apnea (Taketomo, et al. 2005).

✓ Magnesium correction or replacement is gradual. It usually takes a couple of days (Taketomo, et al. 2005).

Case study

Electrolyte overdose

Zach is an 11-month-old patient in the pediatric unit (weighing 7.4 kg). An order was written for Zach to receive calcium chloride, 20 mg/kg (as calcium salt), as a supplement infusion over 60 minutes. Based on his weight, the nurse correctly calculated that Zach was to receive 148 mg. A vial of calcium chloride (10%) was dispensed by the pharmacy. The nurse incorrectly interpreted the concentration of the vial to be 10 mg/ml, rather than 100 mg/ml, resulting in a tenfold overdose. The infant sustained temporary bradycardia and elevated calcium levels, but he eventually recovered.

1. How could this error have been avoided?

2. What processes do you have in place in your institution to prevent errors such as this from occurring?

Chapter 8 | **Cardiovascular medications**

Learning objectives

After reading this chapter, the reader will be able to:

- Recognize why some cardiovascular medications are considered pediatric high-alert medications

- Describe the cardiovascular medications most commonly used in pediatric patients

- Identify at least three ways to prevent errors when administering cardiovascular medications to pediatric patients

Why are cardiovascular medications identified as pediatric high-alert medications?

The cardiovascular system consists of the heart and all of the vessels that provide blood flow to and from the body and lungs. The body depends on the cardiovascular system to operate within a narrow range of normal physiologic parameters. When important cardiovascular parameters—such as blood pressure or heart rate—are above or below the appropriate range, the whole body can be adversely affected. Similarly, the medications that have effects on the cardiovascular system can be used to either decrease or increase those parameters back to a normal range. However, the risk of overshooting the normal range with dosing that is too high can cause significant adverse effects. Their role in maintaining just the right physiologic parameters for such an important organ system is what makes many of the cardiovascular medications pediatric high-alert medications.

Although all organ systems play a vital role in supporting life, the cardiovascular system is the most obvious example: A properly functioning heart is necessary to pump life-sustaining blood throughout the body. Whether they are due to a disease state or simply the aging process, many conditions can cause the heart and cardiovascular system to function at a less than optimal capacity. Fortunately, a number of different medications can be used to augment the cardiovascular system.

Therapeutic options

Cardiovascular medications affect the cardiovascular system in many different ways. They may affect the electrical system (antiarrhythmics), the speed and force of heart contraction (intropes), the degree of vessel contraction and dilation (vasopressors and vasodilators), and the amount of fluid in the body (diuretics). The endpoint of all therapy is appropriate flow of blood throughout the body.

There are numerous drugs that have effects on the cardiovascular system. Although all of the drugs carry some risks for those who receive them, not all cardiovascular medications are considered to be high-risk meds. Those that are fall into the high risk category are the continuous infusion medications including dopamine, dobutamine, milrinone, phenylephrine, isoproterenol, nitroglycerin, nitroprusside, alprostadil, lidocaine, and amiodarone. Some intermittent IV and oral medications antihypertensive agents are also considered high-risk medications.

While this chapter will focus on the cardiovascular agents that are truly high-risk, important safety aspects of other pediatric cardiovascular medications will also be considered.

Who is at risk?

The autonomic system is important in determining the activity of the heart. Many medications, such as dopamine and epinephrine, exert their cardiovascular effects on the heart by activating or blocking autonomic receptors. Therefore, patients who have abnormal autonomic responses—either overactive or underactive—are at a greater risk for medication errors from agents with autonomic activity.

Patients who have congenital heart disease or surgery to correct congenital heart disease may have entirely different hemodynamics and physiologic responses to variations in blood pressure and heart rate. Depending on the type of condition and surgery they have had, they may have an enhanced or reduced response to typical doses of cardiovascular medications. This may put them at risk for adverse effects as the proper patient-specific dosing is determined.

Infections or other disease states can place extra strain on the cardiovascular system and put patients at risk for hemodynamic consequences. In addition, disease states or drugs that affect the structure or function of the cardiovascular system can place patients at increased risk for a weakened or exaggerated response to cardiovascular agents. Patients with poor renal function may accumulate medications that affect the heart, such as milrinone, making it hard to titrate therapy when blood pressure falls or rises suddenly.

The more cardiovascular medications that a patient is on, the more risk there is for the patient. In addition to the risk for more adverse events and direct drug–drug interactions, varying mechanisms can have overlapping or contradictory effects that make titration of a given agent difficult. For example, in the midst of a postop course, a cardiovascular surgery patient may become stabilized on a milrinone and norepinephrine regimen that can cause both vasodilation and vasoconstriction, respectively. However, stopping the vasoconstrictive agent alone may end up causing an imbalance in receptor stimulation and lead to too much vasodilation. Further complicating the adjustment of various agents are the different pharmacokinetic profiles. You would see the effects of stopping or reducing the dose of norepinephrine shortly after you made the adjustment, whereas it may take several hours to see the change in physiologic response after stopping or reducing the dose of milrinone. Intensivists in a monitored setting can successfully make these types of adjustments, but the complexity definitely increases the risk of error.

The use of nonstandardized continuous infusions increases patient risk as well (Larsen 2005). Continuous medication infusions, or drips, can provide patient-specific dosing by one of two methods: rate-based or concentration-based. The concentration-based method keeps the concentration constant and varies the rate to adjust the dose, whereas the rate-based method keeps the rate constant from patient to patient but requires variations in concentration to adjust the dose. The preparation of different concentrations for each different-size patient allows many opportunities for error in the preparation and dispensing of drips. When prescribers have a limited number of concentrations to choose from and pharmacists have a limited number of concentrations to make, the result is increased safety for the patient. This increased safety is further enhanced when the standard concentrations are selected to make what is commercially available. Dopamine, for example, is manufactured as a 1.6 mg/mL concentration that is ready for infusion. Selecting this concentration allows a dopamine drip to be provided to the patient without any further manipulation or dilution in the pharmacy. This approach can also greatly simplify the preparation of dopamine in a code situation.

Pediatric considerations

Epidemiology

The causes of heart failure and arrhythmias are generally very different in children. In adults, heart failure is usually due to the cardiac muscle wearing out from many years of strain. In children, most heart problems are due to congenital heart disease or its repair (Odland 2006). This is also true of arrhythmias. More often than not, an arrhythmia in a child is secondary to cardiovascular surgery or a congenital anomaly in the conducting tissue (Doniger 2006).

Physiology

Pediatric patients tend to control their systemic blood flow by rate rather than by force of contraction. Unlike adults, infants and young children do not have the muscle mass to overcome low blood pressure by increasing the force of cardiac muscle contraction. Therefore, in response to low blood pressure, an infant or child's heart will speed up to accommodate and provide increased blood flow. In addition, children have much more resilient, responsive vessels than adults do. Over time, the elasticity and function of the arteries wear out in adult patients. This can make blood pressure less of an acute concern and easier to control in the pediatric population. Pediatric patient have less sympathetic innervation of the heart, thus requiring higher doses of medications that have their effects on the sympathetic nervous system.

Pharmacokinetics

Because inotropes and other continuous infusion medications are generally short-acting, not much pharmacokinetic variation can be seen between pediatric and adult patients. In intermittent dosing, however, it is not uncommon for children to require a decreased interval for the administration of intermittent medications. This is likely due to faster clearance of the medication by the increased hepatic metabolism found in pediatric patients.

Drug formulations

For drips, the commercially available concentrations are fairly convenient for use in children. Pediatric concentrations are generally the same as or higher than adult concentrations. Although the commercially available ready-to-use concentrations may be too diluted for some pediatric patients, custom-made drips can be made as needed by diluting concentrated forms of the desired drug. The only major drawback to drug formulations for drips is that they often do not come in a convenient volume. For example, the commercially available ready-to-use infusions of dopamine come in a 250 mL bag. There is a risk in hanging a 250 mL bag on a small child whose daily dose may require only 24 mL of the drug. The accidental infusion of the entire bag could easily result in a greater than tenfold overdose, which could be fatal given the high-risk status of continuous infusion cardiovascular drips. Furthermore, the drips provided to infants and small children are often administered using syringe pumps for improved accuracy at lower infusion rates. Even if a standard concentration is available from the manufacturer for a certain drug, the pharmacy must still manipulate that concentration to provide the final product in a syringe. Even the simple process of transferring drugs from one container to another carries a risk for human error that could result in patient harm.

Oral drug formulations of cardiovascular agents are more problematic in children. Most commercially available tablets come in strengths that are too high for pediatric patients, and they are often not in a dosage form that can be conveniently split. To further complicate the issue, very few cardiovascular agents are available in oral liquid dosage forms. Although pharmacies can compound some formulations, the process of making liquid dosage forms is not a simple practice or exact science. Therefore, they introduce another aspect of risk for pediatric patients.

Drug indications

Although different etiologies are behind the need for cardiovascular agents in adults and children, the general indications are the same: hypertension, hypotension, and arrhythmias.

Medical management

One of the biggest differences in the medical management of pediatric patients compared to adults is the lack of available data to guide therapy. Adult cardiovascular medicine is driven by large-scale trials that aim to show mortality benefits for the available therapies. In children, the ability to conduct large clinical trials is not possible. Therefore, much of the medical management is driven by experience rather than by science. This results in different practitioners developing different approaches to treating the same disease states. Although there is some standardization of therapy through published case reports and national meetings, much of pediatric cardiovascular therapy is individualized and quite different from one institution to another, or even from one attending physician to another.

Compliance

The problems with compliance and cardiovascular medications are twofold. First, because many drugs are not available in pediatric formulations, the pediatric patient may be required to take medications that are crushed or formulated into a liquid dosage form. Often, medications that are crushed have a terrible taste that some patients may not be able to tolerate. Even medications that are extemporaneously prepared in sugar solutions are not likely to have the same palatability as commercially manufactured products. Pharmacies can purchase flavoring systems to increase the palatability of compounded dosage forms, but they are expensive and still may not mask the taste of all medications.

The second issue in compliance is due to the long-term, chronic nature of cardiovascular disease in pediatric patients. Some congenital heart patients may need to remain on multiple medications for life. This can be a challenge for young children, particularly in a school setting. As children grow older, they tend to face a different set of challenges as adolescents in that they often lose interest in keeping up with a demanding medication schedule. This is an even greater problem when patients do not notice any particular short-term health benefit of taking their medications. Appropriate discharge counseling and frequent follow-up are important in making sure that patients with long-term medication needs are staying on track with their therapy.

Drug-specific information

Dopamine: The effects of this drug depend on the dose administered—lower doses increase heart rate, and higher doses cause vasoconstriction. Dopamine can be confused with dobutamine, which has different dose-related activity. Using TALLman lettering can help improve the safety and visibility of sound-alike look-alike drugs: Dopamine and DOBUTamine.

Epinephrine: This drug comes in several commercially available concentrations for several different routes of administration that may be easily confused—confirm the concentration before preparing or administering a dose. For intravenous administration, there are two concentrations available that, if confused, can result in a 10-fold error. See Figure 8.1.

As you can see from the table, the ratio strength is inversely proportional to the concentration. Although included on the manufacturer's drug packaging, describing the strength of epinephrine using the ratio strength can be confusing and lead to errors. Therefore, it is recommended that concentration alone be used to describe the strength of epinephrine.

| Figure 8.1 | Intravenous epinephrine dosage forms |

Concentration	Ratio strength	Volume	Packaging
0.1 mg/mL	1:10,000	10 mL	Syringe
1 mg/mL	1:1000	1 mL 30 mL	Ampule Vial

Source: *Reference: Lexi-Comp 2006.*

Norepinephrine: Do not confuse this with epinephrine—it can cause significantly more vasoconstriction. Use of TALLman lettering can improve safety and visibility of sound-alike, look-alike drugs (epinephrine, NORepinephrine).

Phenylephrine: Do not confuse with epinephrine—it can cause significantly more vasoconstriction.

Vasopressin: Dosing recommendations can be confusing and are reported in drug references as units/kg/hour, units/kg/minute, units/minute, milliunits/kg/hour—pay careful attention to dosing units; do NOT abbreviate units with "u" or "U."

Nitroprusside/nitroglycerin: These are look-alike/sound-alike drugs with different side-effect profiles.

Nesiritide: Confusion over small doses (0.01–0.05 mcg/kg/min) may result in a tenfold error (0.1–0.5 mcg/kg/min).

Clonidine: This drug can cause rebound hypertension if it is abruptly discontinued; patches can be difficult to use in children and may easily result in overdoses.

Milrinone: This drug has a longer half-life than other continuous infusions and accumulation in renal failure leads to limited ability to rapidly titrate to effect.

Digoxin: Milligram/microgram confusion in dosing can lead to significant overdoses and severe toxicity; this drug should be dosed in *micro*grams, not milligrams. Dose must be reduced in renal dysfunction or when given in combination with amiodarone. Monitoring of drug levels may be necessary for this narrow therapeutic index drug.

Beta-blockers: can worsen asthma; use caution in infants and children since heart rate is the major way that the immature heart regulates blood pressure.

Nifedipine: This drug can cause dangerously rapid falls in blood pressure when short-acting agents are given orally.

Lidocaine: Drug levels should be monitored to avoid significant toxicity; toxicity can be enhanced in heart or liver failure.

Propafenone: Not available in pediatric dosage form—cutting tablets or extemporaneously preparing this narrow therapeutic drug must be done carefully and as consistently as possible.

Adenosine: Short-half-life (10 seconds) requires fast administration at the IV site closest to the heart

Amiodarone: Multiple drug interactions and significant side effects require careful monitoring during administration of this drug; its extremely long half-life requires consideration for drug interactions and side effects for weeks after therapy.

Alprostadil: Also known as prostaglandin E, or PGE. Do not confuse with other prostaglandin products.

Nursing implications

Administering cardiovascular medications to children pulls into play all aspects of current high-alert medication safety. Although not all cardiovascular mediactions are traditionally considered high-alert medications, their clinical significance, complex calculations and, in many cases, their continuous infusion delivery route makes many of the medications discussed in this chapter at risk for potentially devastating outcomes if errors occur. Initiatives such as CPOE, standard concentrated drips, smartpump technology, and independent double-check systems address the potentially dangerous steps in cardiovascular medication administration and are essential to improving pediatric cardiovascular medication safety.

Administration and safety considerations

✓ Central lines are preferable for continuous infusions.

✓ Many of these drugs are incompatible with other medications commonly used to treat children with cardiac defects, diseases, or disorders. Be familiar with compatibility information prior to any drug administration.

✓ Frequent adjustments or titration is often necessary with these types of medications. Orders for titration should include a starting dose, clinical parameters for titration (such as "maintain MAP 30–40 mmHg"), and maximum drug dose to be titrated to (Bowden & Greenberg, 1998)).

✓ Allow time for drugs to take effect. Avoid becoming caught in a "yo-yo" of titrating too quickly one way and then the other.

✓ Reduce myocardial oxygen consumption by decreasing environmental stressors. Address pain, anxiety, or agitation immediately. Monitor and treat fevers quickly. Promote a supportive, relaxed environment (Hazinski, M., 1991; Slota, M., 2006).

✓ Pediatric emergency equipment, including resuscitation medications and a pediatric-appropriate defibrillator, should be easily accessible.

Monitoring

✓ Set continuous monitor alarms as appropriate. Make sure they are turned *on*.

✓ Check vital signs frequently.

✓ In many instances, continuous EKG and pulse oximetry monitoring is required.

✓ Check the patient's blood pressure. If you are using invasive arterial blood pressure monitoring, verify a cuff BP at least every eight hours or per institutional policy.

✓ Monitor other hemodynamic parameters according to prescribed therapies (central venous pressure, cardiac output, etc.).

✓ Closely monitor the patient's respiratory status.

✓ Blood gas monitoring may be required, according to patient status and prescribed treatment.

✓ Monitor perfusion, accurate intake and output, fluid balance, renal and hepatic function, and electrolytes (Taketomo, et al. 2005)

✓ Monitor IV sites closely. Many of these agents have the potential to cause severe tissue necrosis with extravasation (Taketomo, et al. 2005).

✓ Monitor drug levels as appropriate (e.g., Digoxin levels). (Taketomo, et al. 2005).

Case study

Low–birth weight baby

Molly is a patient in the NICU. She is two days old and has very low birth weight (650 grams). She is receiving a standard concentration of dopamine at 10 mcg/kg/min via a central line. Molly's mom had a fever at the time of Molly's emergency delivery, so Molly is being treated with broad-spectrum antibiotics until her cultures are confirmed. When it is time to administer the next dose of her antibiotic, the nurse notices that the peripheral line she has been using for intermittent medications is puffy and difficult to flush. Because Molly is so small, the nurse cannot easily identify another vein to try for a peripheral IV and decides to administer the antibiotics via the central line. Within two minutes of beginning the antibiotic infusion, the ECG monitor alarm sounds. When she turns around, Molly's nurse notices that Molly's blood pressure is nearly double what it was just a short time ago.

1. What is causing Molly's sudden hypertension?

2. What could have been done to prevent this error?

Case study

Pump safety

Stella is a two year old in the PICU being treated for severe sepsis and cardiomyopathy. She is on a significant number of continuous infusion medications, including dopamine, norepinephrine, and morphine. Because she has required increased titration of the norepinephrine drip, the drip is about to run out, so the nurse calls the pharmacy for a replacement. When the new medication syringe arrives, the nurse checks it against the original order and a second nurse confirms that it is correct as well. The order reads 0.05 mcg/kg/min. The nurse attaches the new medication syringe, sets the pump, and turns away from Stella's bedside. Within minutes Stella's monitors are alarming and the nurse notes that her blood pressure is 148/98. When she checks the infusion that was just started, she notices that the pump is running at 5 mcg/kg/min, not 0.05 mcg/kg/min as ordered.

1. What is causing Stella's sudden hypertension?

2. What could have been done to prevent this error?

3. What systems to you have in place to prevent errors such as the ones described in these two case studies from occurring?

Patient and family education highlights

Inotropic agents:

✓ Most inotropic agents are used exclusively in ICU settings due to the continuous and often complex monitoring that is required.

✓ Digoxin may be used in the ICU, step-down, and general care areas and may even be prescribed for use at home following discharge.

✓ Assess apical pulse before administering Digoxin. Be familiar with the signs and symptoms of Digoxin toxicity (Taketomo, C., et al. 2005).

Antiarrhythmic medications:

✓ Conduct continuous or routine ECG monitoring

✓ Assess PR, QT, and QRS intervals since antiarrythmias can also cause other arrythmias (Slota 2006)

✓ Many antiarrhythmic drugs increase the drug levels of a number of other medications

Antihypertensives:

✓ Follow BP closely, especially before and after medication administration (Taketomo, et al. 2005)

✓ Monitor potassium levels closely when antihypertensive or diuretic medications are part of the medication regimen (Slota 2006)

✓ Keep volume expanders, such as normal saline, readily available in the event that the patient becomes severely hypotensive (Slota 2006)

Many medications exert their effects on the heart and blood vessels. Any medication that affects the flow of blood throughout the body carries some risk. However, only agents that are administered continuously or have significant potential for hemodynamic compromise warrant consideration as a high-risk medication.

Chapter 9 | # Insulin and concentrated dextrose solutions

Learning objectives

After reading this chapter, the reader will be able to:

- Recognize why insulin and concentrated dextrose solutions are considered pediatric high-alert medications

- Describe the insulin and concentrated dextrose solutions most commonly used in pediatric patients

- Identify at least three ways to prevent errors when administering insulin and concentrated dextrose solutions to pediatric patients

Why are insulin and concentrated dextrose solutions identified as pediatric high-alert medications?

Insulin and concentrated dextrose solutions play a significant role in the homeostasis of blood glucose. Errors in dosing, preparation, dispensing, and administration of these medications can result in serious cardiac disturbances, electrolyte imbalances, seizures, coma, and even death (Taketomo, et al. 2005). The Institute for Safe Medication Practices (ISMP) includes medications such as insulin on the list of drugs that have a heightened risk of causing significant patient harm when used in error. Insulin is a potential look-alike, sound-alike medication due to the way it is packaged and to the many different types and concentrations available. If given by mistake, the consequences could be devastating.

Dextrose (d-glucose) is a monosaccharide (simple sugar) similar to electrolytes in that it is often considered to be simply a nutritional product. Although its importance as a macronutrient cannot be ignored, its role in many physiological processes and its risk for patient harm require the same careful attention as any high-risk drug. When referring to the concentration of dextrose in a physiologic context, the term *glucose* or *blood sugar* is generally used.

The body has been designed to operate within a very small window of appropriate glucose concentration (approximately 80–120 mg/dL). Excursions above (hyperglycemia) or below (hypoglycemia) that range can cause significant patient harm. Therefore, it is appropriate to evaluate the safety of agents that can raise or lower serum glucose concentration. Hyperglycemic and hypoglycemic agents are essential to the maintenance of normal blood sugar (euglycemia); yet they can both be the cause of significant clinical problems that can result in considerable morbidity and even death.

The first half of this chapter will deal with dextrose solutions, and the second half will deal with insulin.

Therapeutic options with concentrated dextrose solutions

Simply enough, giving dextrose or glucose (both refer to the same monohydrate) is the way to raise or maintain blood glucose in an acceptable range. Dextrose is prepared and provided to patients in many ways:

- For healthy people who can eat normally, the enteral diet is the source of carbohydrates or complex sugars that are further broken down into glucose

- Glucose tablets and gels are available for diabetic patients who may need a quick boost in blood sugar to overcome an acute episode of hypoglycemia

- In hospitalized patients unable to take enteral nutrition, dextrose-containing fluids or total parenteral nutrition (TPN) are the means of providing the essential sugar

- Lastly, patients who are in emergent need of dextrose can receive intravenous bolus doses of concentrated dextrose

Just as there are many ways to provide dextrose to patients, there are many ways to express appropriate dosing. Whether the term *glucose* or *dextrose* is used, the doses refer to the same amount of carbohydrate. Chewable glucose tablets are dosed in grams. Liquid dosage forms—oral gels, oral liquids, or intravenous liquids—are generally described in terms of a concentration (e.g., 10%) and a corresponding volume. Although the concentration is an important consideration for the site of administration, expressing the dosing in terms of concentration and volume can lead to significant errors.

Case study

TPN therapy

A young patient on home TPN came into the hospital. During the boy's stay, his nutrition plan was to continue on the same TPN order. When the pharmacy obtained the label from the patient's home TPN, a significant mistake was made. The pharmacist interpreted the line "300 mL of 50% dextrose" as a final concentration of 50% dextrose. Even though this is twice as high as the typical maximum concentration of dextrose in a TPN, the bag was made, delivered to the floor, and administered to the patient. This mistake resulted in the patient's death just two days later.

1. What could have prevented this fatal mistake?

2. What safeguards can you implement at your hospital to prevent a similar tragic event from occurring?

Because of the danger of confusing different percentages as illustrated in the above case, it is recommended that only the final concentration to be administered be included on TPN labels (ASPEN 1997). Furthermore, it is recommended that the dose of dextrose on a TPN label be standardized to indicate the amount of the drug in grams/day (ASPEN 1997). The dextrose in TPN solutions is often more precisely defined as a glucose infusion rate in terms of mg/kg/minute of dextrose, but this is often not included on the label.

Who is at risk with concentrated dextrose solutions?

Similar to electrolytes, there is a significantly increased risk for medication errors when intravenous supplementation is required. In an enteral overdose, the body has the opportunity to excrete or distribute the excess glucose before it reaches the critical target end organs, such as the brain. Intravenous products are instilled directly into the veins with faster, less opposed access to the brain. Patients who have diabetes mellitus, impaired glucose tolerance, or a family history of such disease states are more likely to require non-enteral forms of glucose supplementation for periods of acute hypoglycemia. Thus, they are at an increased risk for dextrose-related complications.

A further complication with intravenous dosing is the final concentration for administration. Dextrose comes in a 70% solution for TPN compounding and 50% for emergency bolus infusion, yet the maximum recommended concentration for peripheral infusion is only 10%–12%. In emergencies, concentrations of up to 25% have been used, but the risk of thrombosis, pain, vein irritation, and tissue necrosis increases with increasing concentrations. The dextrose concentration is also a concern in TPN, which is often administered peripherally yet can have dextrose concentrations of up to 30%. Similar to other dextrose infusions, a TPN must not be administered peripherally if the dextrose concentration is higher than 12% (Lexi-Comp 2006).

In addition to the injection site tissue injury caused by high dextrose concentrations, more severe reactions can occur when high dextrose concentrations are infused rapidly. Rapid elevations in serum glucose can cause fluid and electrolyte shifts that result in dehydration, increased serum osmolarity, coma, and even death. Careful adherence to recommended infusion limits in combination with close monitoring of serum glucose, serum osmolarity, and urine glucose can protect patients from such dire consequences (Lexi-Comp 2006).

Patients who have disease states that predispose them to high serum osmolarity (e.g., chronic uremia) and patients who have carbohydrate intolerance are at an even greater risk for adverse outcomes due to rapid dextrose administration (Lexi-Comp 2006).

Pediatric considerations with concentrated dextrose solutions

Epidemiology

Historically, diabetes mellitus was not considered a common problem in pediatric patients. However, an increasing number of young patients are developing type 1 and type 2 diabetes.

Physiology

Children, especially infants and newborns, have increased carbohydrate requirements as part of their natural development and growth. Thus, pediatric patients require higher doses of intravenous dextrose when receiving maintenance fluids or TPN. In addition, children often have significant fluid restrictions that require the use of higher concentrations to provide the clinically necessary dose of dextrose. This increases their risk of local and systemic side effects compared to adults. In addition to the systemic adverse reactions found in adults, infants are also at risk for intracerebral hemorrhage as a result of rapid administration of high concentrations of dextrose (Lexi-Comp 2006).

Drug formulations

Because pediatric patients often require higher doses and less fluid volume, concentrated formulations make pediatric dosing easier but increase risks for fatal overdoses. Therefore, it is important to treat concentrated dextrose solutions like concentrated electrolytes and only store them in the pharmacy. The one exception is the 50% dextrose syringe that can be stored with the emergency medications in the nursing unit. Another way to protect pediatric patients from concentrated electrolytes is to build concentration limits into the automated ordering, dispensing, and administration programs used in the hospital. If the pharmacy computer system has dextrose concentrations built into dose-checking software, this adds another layer of safety for patients.

Drug indications

In 20%–40% of pediatric patients, their initial presentation of diabetes is in diabetic ketoacidosis. Diabetic ketoacidosis is a condition which will require intravenous dextrose solutions as part of the corrective therapy. Similar to adults, patients who needs caloric intake from fluids or have hypoglycemia should receive dextrose solutions. The appropriate concentration will depend on the patient's clinical status and route of administration.

Medical management

The adult limits for peripheral concentration, central concentration, and maximum rates of infusion apply to pediatric patients as well.

Compliance

Children rarely need to take oral agents to increase glucose, but tolerability is not likely to be as much of a problem due to the sweet taste of oral glucose tablets and liquid glucose. Intravenous administration may be affected by the difficulties in obtaining adequate venous access in small pediatric patients. Given that children often require higher concentrations to meet their increased glucose requirements, central access may be needed more often to allow for safe administration.

Drug-specific information

Given the variety of dangers associated with intravenous dextrose solutions, appropriate steps should be taken to protect patients from accidental overdoses:

- Although the concentration is an appropriate part of the orders for intravenous dextrose, each order should include a weight-based and final dose in grams, *not* in milliliters.

- The dextrose concentration on a TPN order and label should reflect the final concentration to be administered, *not* the concentration used in preparation.

- The dextrose dose on a TPN order and label should specify a weight-based and total daily dose in grams, *not* per liter of solution.

- Concentrations of dextrose should be standardized as much as clinically possible to enhance the safety of the preparation process. Furthermore, all preparation of dextrose-containing fluids should take place in a pharmacy under a sterile hood.

- Concentrations of dextrose stored on floors and units should be as limited as possible and only in concentrations of 10% or less.

- Concentrated dextrose (50%) for emergency use should only be kept in locked storage cabinets where it cannot be routinely accessed. If possible, the storage of concentrated dextrose on units should be limited to code carts and other emergency storage areas.

- Peer double-checks of dextrose concentrations are another way to add safety to the use of this high-risk medication.

Nursing implications with concentrated dextrose solution

Administration of concentrated dextrose solution in pediatrics relies on all aspects of high-alert medication safety.

Administration and safety considerations: Concentrated dextrose

✓ Dextrose solutions >12.5% must be administered via a central line only; dextrose solutions ≤12.5% can be safely infused via a peripheral IV line but must be monitored closely (per institutional policy) (Taketomo et al. 2005; Young, and Mangum 2007).

✓ Clearly label all medication syringes or IV fluid bags.

✓ Clearly mark tubing, including at connection ports closest to the patient.

✓ Avoid rapid infusion of hypertonic solutions.

✓ Use with caution in premature infants, as rapid changes in osmolarity may produce profound effects on the brain (Taketomo, et al. 2005).

✓ Stock dextrose solutions should be stored separately from other IV solutions and clearly marked according to dextrose concentration (IHI).

✓ Do not store highly concentrated dextrose in patient care areas. (IHI).

✓ Consider locking highly concentrated dextrose solutions, similar to the way narcotics are stored, in pharmacy areas (IHI).

Monitoring

✓ Most adverse effects are associated with excessive dosage concentration, or rate of infusion (Taketomo, et al. 2005).

✓ Monitor blood glucose, urine glucose, serum electrolytes, intake and output, and daily caloric intake (kcal/kg/day).

Patient and family education highlights

✓ Update the child and parents or caregivers on the plan of care

✓ If frequent blood glucose monitoring is necessary, involve the child and family in ways that are appropriate for the child's age, developmental level, and acuity of illness

✓ Teach children, if appropriate for their age and developmental level, as well as parents or care-givers the signs and symptoms of hypoglycemia

Case study

IV bolus

Charlie is a 13-year-old admitted to the ED with a ruptured appendix. The ED staff and the pediatric surgeon have evaluated him, and he is on his way to the operating room for emergency surgery. Before leaving the ED, the pediatric surgeon calls, and he requests that Charlie receive a fluid bolus of lactated ringers (LR), 20 ml/kg, over 15 minutes. Charlie's nurse is busy, so a colleague offers to start Charlie's bolus. The nurse introduces himself to Charlie, tells him what he is going to do, and sets the IV infusion pump to run the bolus. When the bolus is complete, the pump alarm sounds and Charlie's nurse returns to silence the alarm. At that time, he notices that his colleague did not change the IVF, and instead of giving Charlie a bolus of LR, he bo-lused Charlie with the dextrose and electrolyte solution that was hanging as Charlie's maintenance fluids.

1. What potential consequences could result from this type of error?

2. How could this error have been prevented?

3. What processes are in place in your institution to prevent errors like this from occurring?

Therapeutic options with insulin

Considerably more options are available for lowering blood glucose than for raising it. For oral agents alone, there are seven different classes and 15 different antidiabetic agents.

These agents are generally reserved for use in type 2 diabetes mellitus, where insulin secretion is limited relative to the need for glucose utilization. Because the development of type 2 diabetes in children is a relatively new phenomenon, very little information is available to guide the use of these agents in children (NDEP 2004, Gaylor 2004). Lack of experience in pharmacokinetics, dosing, and anticipated side effects is a significant risk factor for using oral antidiabetics in children. Aside from the limitation of incomplete information, nothing specifically sets these agents apart as high-risk meds. Because their roles are to augment and enhance natural insulin secretion, they do not have the potential to cause sudden, significant drops in blood sugar like the insulin products do.

The landscape of insulin agents has changed over the years as well. No longer available are pork and bovine products—all insulins are recombinant human or analogue products. Several newer agents have also come to market recently, including an inhaled form of insulin. This form has several limitations and is not currently a feasible dosage form for pediatric patients. Therefore, the focus of the rest of this chapter will be on parenteral insulin products.

One of the most important considerations in choosing an insulin regimen is the pharmacokinetics of the insulin product. Rapid-acting (lispro, aspart, glulisine) or short-acting (regular) insulins should be given around meals. Intermediate-acting (isophane, lente) or longer-acting (ultralente, detemir, glargine) insulins should be used for basal daytime coverage. It is essential that the patient or patient's caregiver understand the importance of timing the insulin dose with meals. If a short-acting insulin is given and the patient does not eat a meal shortly after administration, the patient's blood glucose could drop to dangerously low levels.

Ease of administration is also a consideration in choosing a dosing regimen. If a regimen is selected that contains five daily injections, it is important to make sure the patient will be able to keep up with that regimen consistently. It would be better to select a less ambitious regimen that the patient can use consistently. Alternatively, use of the newer longer-acting agents can also help limit the number of daily injections needed to achieve basal insulin coverage throughout the day.

Cost will be an issue when selecting a regimen, but this is more of an outpatient issue. However, it is still important to verify that the intended regimen is reasonable for patients to obtain. If they have to cut corners on dosing or skip certain parts of their regimen for financial reasons, it is imperative to design the best clinical regimen that patients can afford.

A key safety issue with any insulin regimen is proper use of the term *Units*. If "u" or "U" is used instead, it could result in a tenfold error in dosing. For example, a handwritten dose of "5U regular insulin SQ with meals" could easily be misread as 50 units—a tenfold overdose. Even though the word units does not appear, that may not register in the mind of the busy pharmacist or nurse who is busy multi-tasking while reading the order.

Who is at risk with insulin?

Determining a patient's initial insulin requirements can be difficult. Therefore, newly diagnosed patients are at risk for receiving too much or too little insulin when they are first started on therapy. On the other hand, patients who have a long history of diabetes may have other concomitant disease states and associated medications that may make the use of insulin more difficult. These patients are also at risk for medication errors that may lead to blood glucose levels outside the desired range.

Really severe patients may require very high insulin doses that are best administered with a more concentrated solution, U-500. However, this insulin product, which is five times more concentrated, can cause much confusion in dosing, especially when a patient comes into the hospital setting. For example, a patient may be on a dose of 125 units of insulin. Using a typical insulin syringe that is calibrated for 100 unit/mL insulin, the patient has been trained to draw up to the 25 unit mark. Because U-500 insulin is 5 times more concentrated than 100 unit/mL insulin, drawing up the U-500 insulin to the 25 unit mark actually provides the correct dose of 125 units. However, the patient may come into the hospital and simply state that their dose as 25 units because that is what the syringe shows. This can lead to significant underdosing if it is not clear to the hospital staff that the patient is using U-500 insulin at home.

Patients with complex regimens or who were started on insulin without proper education are at an increased risk for errors as well. Many insulin regimens can result in four or five daily injections (DeWitt 2003). To simplify this, some short- and intermediate-acting agents can be mixed together. However, mixing can lead to inappropriate dosing of one or both agents. In addition, patients may try to mix certain agents that are not compatible and therefore reduce the effectiveness of their therapy.

Patients who have inconsistent meals and poor eating habits are at increased risk for adverse effects from insulin therapy. This is particularly true if they do not adjust their insulin doses to account for their variability in nutrition intake.

There are many drugs that can cause hyperglycemia or hypoglycemia as a side effect. When a diabetic—particularly a diabetic that requires insulin therapy—is on an concomitant medication that can lead to fluctuations in blood glucose, that places the patient at an increased risk for an adverse drug event. As much as possible, medications should be avoided that can raise or lower blood sugar. However, sometimes a patient with a concomitant disease state may not be able to avoid taking medications that affect blood sugar. For example, a diabetic with hypertension may have responded best to enalapril, a medication that can cause a decrease in blood sugar (Lexi-Comp 2006). When it is in the patient's best interest to continue a medication that affects blood sugar control, careful monitoring of the patient's blood sugar is even more important.

Pediatric considerations with insulin

Epidemiology

Although the overall incidence of diabetes is higher in adults, there is a rapid rise in the incidence of diabetes in children (DeWitt 2003, Gaylor 2004, Alemzadeh 2004, Hirsch 2005). The two age groups that have the highest incidence of diabetes are children five to seven years of age and adolescents entering puberty (Alemzadeh 2004).

Physiology

In children, an autoimmune process can lead to destruction of pancreatic cells and loss of insulin secretion (Alemzadeh 2004). Adults can experience insensitivity to the insulin that is secreted or a reduction in insulin secretion as the pancreatic function declines with overuse.

Drug formulations

The same formulations used in adults work well for children. Some smaller doses may be difficult to draw up accurately due to the highly concentrated adult formulations, but generally this is not an issue for subcutaneous dosing.

Drug indications

Type 1 diabetes mellitus, characterized by lack of insulin secretion, is more common in children. Type 2 diabetes mellitus, characterized by a decreased sensitivity to insulin, is more common in adults. In recent years, however, there has been an unfortunate trend of type 2 diabetes developing in more and more adolescents and children (Gaylor 2004, NDEP 2004).

Medical management

Children typically require higher insulin doses than adults (Williams 2004). Higher doses are also needed during puberty (Williams 2004). These changes in insulin requirements with age can make the maintenance of euglycemia difficult in children. In addition, as residual pancreatic function goes away, there will be a need for an increased insulin dose.

Compliance

Compliance can be hard enough with oral medications, but daily injections of insulin on top of finger sticks for monitoring make compliance with diabetic treatment very difficult for children. Thorough, individualized patient and caregiver treatment is essential to improving compliance and making the most out of insulin therapy. Once a patient is stabilized on a good regimen, it is possible to transition to an insulin pump (Williams 2004). The patient must wear or carry this device at all times, but at least it eliminates the need for multiple daily injections.

Drug-specific information with insulin

Regular insulin: The only insulin that can be given intravenously; can cause hypoglycemia if no food is eaten within 30 minutes of administration; prolonged effect may cause some late hypoglycemia even if initially given with food.

Lispro, aspart, glulisine insulins: Rapid-acting; food *must* be given before or shortly after administration to avoid hypoglycemia.

Isophane (NPH), lente, ultralente insulins: Slower onset precludes use for mealtime coverage; longer-acting, but less peak effect than regular insulin.

Glargine insulin: Long-acting, not for use in mealtime coverage; effects can last 24 hours.

Detemir insulin: Not quite as long-acting as glargine; usually requires twice-daily dosing.

Premixed insulins: Intermediate-acting/short-acting in combinations of 70/30 or 50/50. These insulins provide less ability to titrate and poor lunchtime coverage. They can be a way to simplify an insulin regimen for a patient who cannot mix multiple insulins or tolerate more than two injections per day.

Source: *DeWitt 2004, Hirsch 2005, Lexi-Comp 2006.*

Nursing implications with insulin

Insulin-related errors are well documented throughout the safety literature. As a result, numerous safety recommendations exist to decrease insulin-related errors within healthcare organizations. Insulin safety begins in the hospital but must continue when children and their families are on their own at home. Nurses must help children and families learn the effect of insulin and the motor skills involved when administering injections, as well as safe insulin preparation, handling, and storage habits.

Administration and safety considerations with insulin

✓ Store insulin and heparin vials in separate storage areas to avoid look-alike vials (IHI).

✓ Be cautious: Some of the insulin types have sound-alike names, which can lead to accidental mix-ups (such as Humulin® and Humalog®).

✓ A pharmacist should review all orders for insulin prior to administration, except in an emergency (IHI).

✓ A limited number of standard concentrations should be used for insulin infusions (IHI, Joint Commission NPSG 2007).

✓ All insulin infusions will undergo an independent double-check prior to dispensing and prior to administration (Joint Commission NPSG 2007).

✓ Only *regular* insulin can be given via IV or IM (Taketomo, et al. 2005).

✓ *Do not* administer other IVP and intermittent medications via lines containing continuous insulin infusions. This will result in an inadvertent bolus of insulin.

✓ When mixing regular insulin with other preparations, draw the regular insulin into the syringe *first* (Taketomo, et al. 2005).

✓ More than 50 other medications interact with insulin and may result in either increased or decreased hypoglycemic effects (Taketomo, et al. 2005). Refer to pediatric drug references for additional compatibility information.

✓ Because absorption may vary, insulin dosing should be based on the effect and not solely on the insulin dose listed in reference books (Taketomo, et al. 2005).

Monitoring

✓ Monitor blood sugar according to treatment plan and institutional policies.

✓ Monitor urine sugar and acetone, serum electrolytes, and hemoglobin A.

Patient and family education highlights with insulin

Newly diagnosed diabetics will have a lot to learn about the disease and about insulin treatment. Use the child-friendly and developmentally appropriate methods described in previous chapters to teach children and families about blood glucose monitoring and SQ injections.

✓ If a child is going home using more than one type of insulin, teach the family tips for preventing insulin mix-up errors at home (IHI).

✓ Follow manufacturers' guidelines for storage of insulin products, as they can vary depending on the preparation.

✓ Do not change insulin type without a physician's approval (Taketomo, et al. 2005).

✓ Educate the child and family or caregivers on the signs and symptoms of hypo- and hyperglycemia, insulin preparation and administration, diet, exercise, blood glucose monitoring, and other necessary information related to the disease process and medical management protocol (Taketomo, et al. 2005).

Chapter 10 | Neuromuscular blocking agents

Learning objectives

After reading this chapter, the reader will be able to:

- Recognize why neuromuscular blockers (NMB) are considered a pediatric high-alert medication

- Describe the NMBs most commonly used in pediatric patients

- Identify at least three ways to prevent errors when administering NMBs to pediatric patients

Why are NMBs identified as pediatric high-alert medications?

The Institute for Safe Medication Practices (ISMP) has identified NMB medications as a group of substances that pose significant risk of causing devastating and often fatal harm when used in error (Taketomo, C., et al. 2005). NMBs are often used as an adjunct to general anesthesia and to paralyze a patient temporarily during mechanical ventilation. NMB administration results in paralysis of all skeletal muscles, including the diaphragm. Therefore, an error in storage, dosing, preparation, or administration of an NMB can result in severe respiratory deterioration and even death (ISMP 2005).

NMBs are commonly known among healthcare professionals as paralytics. Given the negative connotation of the term *paralytic*, it is wise to avoid using this term when discussing medications around a patient's friends and family. They may misunderstand the term and be concerned about the safety or quality of care their loved one is receiving.

Case study

Misplaced NMB

The emergency department was running over capacity all night, including multiple traumas and a transport on the way. In preparation for the incoming patient, the ED charge nurse decided to pull up the rapid sequence intubation medications. She carefully labeled each syringe and placed them near the intubation equipment. While drawing up the last medication, pancuronium, a colleague called from the hallway that he needed help with a patient. She quickly put down the syringe in her hand and ran to help. While out of the room, the incoming transport arrived. He was a 15-year-old with multiple injuries. Fortunately, the patient was breathing on his own and did not require intubation. A peripheral IV was started for fluids, and upon flushing the IV, the patient suddenly stopped breathing and required emergency intubation. In an attempt to determine what had happened to him, the charge nurse entered the room and noticed the medication syringe she had left on the table was gone. When she asked what had happened to it, her colleague responded that they assumed it was a flush and used it when starting the patient's IV. The child required mechanical ventilation for nearly 14 hours, before the pancuronium effect completely wore off and he was able to breath on his own.

1. How could this error have been prevented?

2. What processes are in place in your institution to prevent errors like this from occurring?

NMBs are often grouped with sedatives and analgesics when it comes to classifying the drug. This is likely due to its concomitant use and shared therapeutic endpoint of keeping patients calm and appropriately motionless. However, there are major differences in how these medications work and how they are used clinically. Furthermore, the risks of therapy with NMBs are profound enough to warrant individualized attention as a unique class.

Therapeutic options

There are two classes of NMBs with directly opposite mechanisms of inducing paralysis. The first class comprises depolarizing NMBs, of which succinylcholine is the only therapeutic option. This agent mimics the depolarizing action of acetylcysteine but in a sustained manner that essentially tires out the muscle fibers. It is generally limited to use in intubation procedures due to its fast onset and short duration of action. The second class, nondepolarizing NMBs, block the normal action of acetylcysteine on muscle contraction, thus rendering the muscle fibers paralyzed. A number of agents are available in this class, including cisatracurium, pancuronium, rocuronium, and vecuronium. Selection of the appropriate agent will depend on the time to onset, duration of action, clearance, adverse reactions, and cost.

It is important to keep in mind that none of the NMBs provide any amount of sedation, anesthesia, or amnesia. Therefore, it is very important that they never be used alone. To receive NMBs without adequate sedation and analgesia is a terrifying experience for patients. Not only do they experience undue pain and anxiety but they also are not able to communicate their needs verbally or physically due to their paralyzed state.

Who is at risk?

Because NMBs result in paralysis of all muscles—including the diaphragm—they cause respiratory arrest at therapeutic doses. It is imperative that a patient be intubated or undergoing a procedure for intubation before a dose of an NMB is ordered or given. In a realistic sense, any patient that is not intubated is at risk for adverse effects from the accidental administration of an NMB. You can take measures to protect nonintubated patients from accidental administration of an NMB. For example, all paralytics should be discontinued from patients' profiles as soon as they are extubated. It is not uncommon for PRN medications—including NMBs—to be left on a profile long after the patient's need for the medication has passed. Removing floor stock supplies of NMBs is also a safety measure to protect nonintubated patients. Any delivery of NMBs to an ICU should be done on a patient-specific basis. If a supply of NMBs is necessary on a given unit, it should be clearly labeled and bagged in such a way as to bring attention to the risk of respiratory arrest when given to a nonintubated patient. It should also be isolated in a locked cabinet to avoid accidental selection from a medication drawer with multiple drugs.

Patients with concomitant disease states are at risk for additional complications from NMBs. For example, patients who have sustained a significant burn injury experience prolonged effects from NMBs due to reduced plasma cholinesterase activity (Brandom 2002). In addition, those with recent muscle injuries are more sensitive to myopathy and hyperkalemia associated with succinylcholine use (Brandom 2002).

Patients who are on long-term or continuous neuromuscular blockade are at increased risk for muscular atrophy as well as third-space accumulation of fluids (Brandom 2002). Ways to avoid these complications include physical therapy (if appropriate for the patient's overall clinical situation) and temporary cessation of the continuous infusion with careful monitoring to prevent unnecessary movements.

Pediatric considerations

Epidemiology

NMBs outside of the usual uses for general anesthesia and tracheal intubation are more likely in pediatric patients compared to adults because infants and children may be more prone to agitation or may not be able to comprehend the need to remain still after surgery (Fisher 1999).

Physiology

The diaphragm and the muscles innervated by the facial nerve are more resistant to neuromuscular blockade than the hand or foot. As a result, the use of peripheral nerve stimulation, or Train of Four, does not correlate well with clinical suppression of respiration (Brandom 2002).

Pharmacokinetics

Onset of action is faster in children than in adults (Brandom 2002). The volume of distribution reflects the extracellular fluid volume; therefore, the volume of distribution is larger in infants compared to children (Brandom 2002). This leads to an increase in clearance for drugs that are cleared via enzymatic activity in the blood (succinylcholine, cisatracurium). In drugs cleared by liver metabolism and renal excretion, there is a longer half-life in infants compared to children (Brandom 2002). For example, the clearance of rocuronium is slower in infants than in children. Overall, the increased extracellular fluid in infants results in lower concentrations of drug in the blood than children and adults when the same weight-based doses are used. This decrease in drug concentration in the blood is offset by an increased sensitivity to NMB's in infants (Fisher 1999). As infants grow and the percentage of total body water decreases, the drug concentrations will rise to adult levels sometime after the first year of life (Fisher 1999).

Drug formulations

When IV access is not available, intramuscular (IM) administration in children is possible but not optimal. The best agent for IM injection is rocuronium. Some of the available agents, like pancuronium and cisatracurium, contain benzyl alcohol—a preservative that should be avoided in neonates (Lexi-Comp 2006).

Drug indications

In addition to use in intubation and general anesthesia, pediatric patients may receive NMBs to promote healing of delicate surgical areas that may be disrupted by intentional or unintentional movement. NMBs may also be used to reduce the physiologic stresses of dysynchronous breathing in critically ill patients (Fisher 1999).

Medical management

The potency of all NMBs varies according to the patient's age. NMBs are more potent in infants than in children and are less potent in children than in adults (Brandom 2002).

There are two approaches to dosing NMBs: continuous infusion and intermittent administration. Due to the relatively short duration of NMBs, they are routinely given as a continuous infusion in adults. Because pediatric patients tend to have a faster onset and a prolonged clearance of the drug, it is possible to provide adequate paralysis with intermittent, as-needed dosing. This does require close monitoring for the proper time to administer the next dose, but it can reduce the consequences of prolonged or excessive paralysis.

There are several agents that can act as NMB reversal agents: neostigmine, pyridostigmine, and edrophonium. Generally, these are used as reversal agents after surgery; however, they also may be used as antidotes in the event of a adverse drug event or medication error (Lexi-Comp 2006, Duncan 1999).

Compliance

Histamine release (most common with succinylcholine, mivacurium, and atracurium) can lead to significant hypotension and tachycardia (Brandom 2002). Anaphylactic and anaphylactoid reactions are also common and can limit the use of certain agents. Bronchospasms due to the cholinergic (M2 receptor) activity in children may further limit the number of drugs that may be safely given to children (Brandom 2002).

Drug-specific information

Succinylcholine: nonreversible; significantly increased risk of side effects, including malignant hyperthermia; requires refrigeration

Atracurium: look-alike, sound-alike potential with cisatracurium, but significantly different dosing, onset of action, and duration of action; significant side-effect profile including hypotension, increased respiratory secretions, and seizures (with drug accumulation)

Cisatracurium: look-alike, sound-alike potential with atracurium, but significantly different dosing, onset of action, and duration of action

Doxacurium: look-alike, sound-alike possibility with doxycycline; slow onset of action; long, unpredictable duration of action

Mivacurium: prolonged duration in renal or hepatic failure; hypotension and tachycardia related to histamine release

Pancuronium: significant cardiovascular effects; active metabolites; prolonged duration in renal or hepatic failure

Rocuronium: long, unpredictable duration of action; refrigeration required after 30 days

Vecuronium: active metabolites; dose reduction needed in hepatic failure

Source: *Lexi-Comp 2006, Micromedex.*

Nursing implications

Neuromuscular blocking agents are most often used in ICU, OR, or emergency department settings. They are integrated into the child's care when it is necessary that the child remain completely still. As described earlier, NMBs do not provide sedation or analgesia, so it is imperative that physicians, nurses, and the entire care team ensure comfort measures are also provided and that pain and sedation levels are continuously monitored and treated.

Administration and safety considerations

- ✓ Only experienced clinicians should be administering and monitoring patients receiving NMB agents (McKenry and Salerno, 2003).

- ✓ NMB agents should be administered only after adequate sedation and pain medication have been initiated. A combination of opioid analgesics and benzodiazepines are common—opioids so that the child does not feel pain and benzodiazepines for their amnesic affects. (Hazinski 1991).

- ✓ Administer NMBs to *ventilated* patients only (ISMP 2005).

- ✓ Use some sort of eye lubrication.

- ✓ Implement developmentally appropriate safety interventions during treatment with NMBs, including appropriate use of bed side rails or crib rails.

- ✓ Pediatric emergency equipment should be easily accessible in any area where NMB agents are being used.

- ✓ It is not uncommon in ED, ICU, and OR settings to reconstitute a vial containing an NMB agent and use it repeatedly for intermittent dosing. This is a potentially dangerous practice, as the vial could be confused for another look-alike medication.

- ✓ Some NMB agents cause increased oral secretions as well as thickening of secretions. Suction should always be available (Young & Mangum, 2007).

- ✓ Provide frequent change of position and document changes to minimize skin breakdown.

Case study

Sound-alike medications

A physician requested Narcan (nalaxone) for a newly extubated baby to reverse the effects of fentanyl, which the baby had been receiving prn post-operatively. The nurse did not recognize the drug that was being asked for because she was used to referring to it by its generic name. She intended to ask a coworker for Narcan's generic name, but in the chaos of trying to stabilize the baby, asked her coworker for the generic name for Norcuron instead. Her coworker told her that Norcuron was vecuronium, which the nurse then administered. The child arrested, and following the reintubation, remained mechanically ventilated for more than three days.

1. How could this error have been avoided?

2. What processes does your institution have in place to prevent an error like this from occurring?

3. How might you approach explaining to this patient's family what happened?

Monitoring

✓ Dosing and titration are based on the child's clinical response (Taketomo, C., et al. 2005).

✓ A peripheral nerve stimulator can be used to monitor the level of sedation (Taketomo, C., et al. 2005).

✓ Patients should be on continuous ECG, capnography, pulse oximetry, and blood pressure monitoring (Taketomo, et al. 2005).

✓ Monitor and document (per institutional policy) sedation level as well as pain assessment.

✓ Common side effects associated with NMB administration are most often related to the concurrent administration of opioid analgesics. These include:

- Bradycardia

- Hypotension

- Tachycardia

- Hypertension

Patient and family education highlights

✓ Prepare the parent(s) or caregivers for what is going to happen once the NMB is administered. Do the same prior to discontinuing the medication.

✓ Provide families with things they can do to support the child. Although the child is heavily sedated as well as paralyzed, parents often feel they need to "do something." Give them tasks that will not disturb the child, but will allow them to parent in a small but meaningful way:

- Teach parents how to read their child's small cues, such as change in heart rate or oxygen saturations, to gauge how well their activities are being tolerated

- Sing quietly to the child

- Tell a story, or read from a book

- Play soft music

- Assist with gentle range of motion when appropriate (Bowden and Smith-Greenberg 2008)

- Assist in turning and repositioning the child when appropriate

✓ Assure parents or caregivers that the child is being kept comfortable while he or she is medically paralyzed.

Although often overlooked as a class, NMBs are definitely a high-risk medication in that therapeutic doses can be fatal if simply given to the wrong patient or at the wrong time. Failing to recognize the unique aspects of this drug or simply considering NMBs to be "sedative-like" makes the potential for error even more likely. A proactive approach to limiting the potential for accidental administration should be in place at every hospital that stocks neuromuscular blockers.

Chapter 11 | Pediatric pain and sedation medications

Learning objectives

After reading this chapter, the reader will be able to:

- Recognize why some medications used to treat pediatric pain and provide sedation are considered pediatric high-alert medications

- Describe the classes of medication used for pain and sedation treatment in pediatric patients

- Identify at least three ways to prevent errors when administering pain medications to pediatric patients

- List at least five common safety components of any pediatric sedation program

Why are some pediatric pain and sedation agents identified as high-alert medications?

The Institute for Safe Medication Practices (ISMP) along with The Joint Commission has identified many of the medications used to provide pain management or sedation to children as a group of substances that pose significant risk of causing devastating and often fatal harm when used in error (Taketomo, C., et al. 2005). An opiate (morphine) was among the six medications on the first list of high-alert medications published by the ISMP in 1989. According to the ISMP, opiates are still among the most frequent high-alert medications to cause patient harm (Smetzer 1998; ISMP).

Central nervous system (CNS) depression is a considerable side effect of these medications. Errors in the ordering, preparation, dispensing, administration, or monitoring of patients receiving these medications can result in damaging outcomes and even death.

The treatment of pain and agitation goes hand in hand, yet pain and agitation are unique entities. Understanding how these two therapeutic concepts are similar yet different is essential to providing safe relief of agitation and pain.

As always, a good place to start is to sort out the definitions of commonly used words (AAP 2001; Rodriguez 2002):

- **Pain:** a subjective experience that involves physiologic, psychological, behavioral, developmental, and situational factors

- **Anxiety:** an emotional state of uneasiness and apprehension

- **Agitation:** a state of anxiety accompanied by motor restlessness

- **Analgesia:** a deadening or absence of pain, without the loss of consciousness

- **Sedation:** a reduction of anxiety, stress, irritability, or excitement

Although they are different by definition, a closer look at the pathophysiology of pain, anxiety, and agitation shows that they are closely linked. The pain that a patient experiences can lead to anxiety and agitation. Furthermore, anxiety and agitation can cause an increased perception of pain (Tang 2005). Thus, pain and anxiety feed off each other and get progressively worse if each is not adequately treated.

Therapeutic options

The overlap in the pathophysiology is also seen in the treatment of pain and anxiety. Analgesics are medications that are used to treat pain, and sedatives are medications that are used to treat anxiety and agitation. Some medications have both sedative and analgesic properties (Tobias 1999).

When selecting a medication, it is very important to consider its range of effect. If a sedative drug is used in a patient during a painful procedure, the child may still experience pain despite appearing calm. In addition to unnecessarily experiencing pain during this procedure, the patient will also experience the physiologic effects of pain on blood pressure and metabolic response (Chambliss 1997). It is also likely that the patient will have increased anxiety during future procedures or physician encounters as a result of having previously experienced pain during a procedure. If a pure analgesic is used for a pediatric procedure, the increased anxiety experienced by the patient while awake during the procedure can lead to an emotionally painful experience and a greater likelihood of anxiety or agitation during future procedures.

Benzodiazepines (midazolam, lorazepam) and barbiturates (phenobarbitol, pentobarbital) are the most common classes of sedatives. Additional sedative agents include propofol, haloperidol, diphenhydramine, chloral hydrate, and etomidate. Opioids (fentanyl, morphine), alpha-2 agonists (clonidine, dexmedetomidine), and the general anesthetic ketamine are all agents with sedative-analgesic properties. Lastly, non-steroidal anti-inflammatory drugs (ibuprofen, ketorolac), local anesthetics (lidocaine, bupivacaine), aspirin, and acetaminophen are agents that only provide pain relief.

Who is at risk?

Overdoses—whether they are oral or intravenous—pose a risk for patients. The biggest concern in overdoses of sedatives and analgesics is respiratory depression. With chronic dosing, patients develop tolerance not only to the effects of sedatives and analgesics but also to the side effects. Therefore, a patient who has no history of sedative or analgesic use is at greatest risk for developing respiratory depression. Patients who have disease states that compromise respiratory function are also at an increased risk for respiratory depression from sedative and analgesic medications. This even includes patients who have sleep apnea.

The more medications that are used to achieve sedation, the greater the risk of respiratory depression and other side effects. This is especially true when multiple agents with different mechanisms of action are used, such as opiates and benzodiazepines.

CNS depression, or sedation, is also a concern with sedatives and analgesics. This is a greater concern in an outpatient setting where individuals may try to carry on normal activities such as driving or working while taking medications that can significantly impair their decision-making and reaction time.

Another outpatient concern is the addition of alcoholic beverages to sedatives and analgesics. Alcoholic beverages further impair the CNS, and the combination of several mechanisms of CNS depression can lead to significant adverse effects.

Pediatric considerations

Epidemiology

Due to the close relationship of anxiety and pain, children have a tendency to experience more pain than adults. Unfamiliar situations and people, noisy machines, separation from parents, bad memories of previous medical experiences, and disturbances in sleep-wake cycles are situational factors that may lead children to experience greater pain than adults in a similar situation. Although adults can also experience increased pain due to situational or emotional factors, it is more common in children due to a child's inability to comprehend what is going on in the unfamiliar setting. Children are also less likely to be able to communicate their concerns and needs, giving them less control and a reduced ability to meet their own needs (Kaushal 2001; McPhillips 2005). Nonverbal children are at an even greater disadvantage because their only means of communicating is nonspecific crying.

Physiology

Historically, there was a popular concept that children—especially infants and neonates—experienced less pain than adults. This has recently been refuted by new information that supports an increased number of pain receptors in newborns, making it likely that they actually experience more pain than adults (Anand 2001).

Pharmacokinetics

Absorption of morphine through the immature gastrointestinal tract is thought to be increased. The decreased renal elimination in neonates may make them more susceptible to the prolonged effects of various sedatives and analgesics. The increased metabolism often found in children can increase or decrease the effect of drugs. For example, drugs eliminated by hepatic metabolism (methadone) will be cleared faster in pediatric patients and may require increased dosing, whereas drugs activated by hepatic metabolism (codeine) may require a decreased dose compared to adult patients.

Drug formulations

Specialized dosage forms such as fentanyl patches and lozenges are *not* appropriate for most pediatric patients for several reasons. First, these are generally designed for use in patients receiving large amounts of opiates, so the available strengths are often much too high in terms of dosage for a pediatric patient. Second, small pediatric patients may receive a disproportionate amount of the drug from topical dosage form based on the pharmacokinetic differences between adults and children. Third, the lozenge is a difficult dose to titrate in a pediatric patient, and there is concern that a young patient may inappropriately chew the entire lozenge and accidentally overdose him or herself if not constantly monitored. Fourth, a high-risk medication that resembles candy has the potential to blur the lines between medication and food for young patients. Even if the dose is administered appropriately, it may create dangerous habits in children who may curiously try other medications that they find lying around.

Drug indications

There are no major differences in the indications for using sedatives and analgesics in children, other than a potentially lower threshold for using an analgesic for a procedure that is considered to be "painless."

Medical management

Children often require less sedation initially and more sedation as they recover (Bhatt-Mehta 1998). The early decrease may have to do with less need during procedures due to pharmacokinetic differences. The increased sedation during recovery may be due to an increased rate of developing tolerance in children or simply due to the stronger connection between anxiety and pain in the pediatric population.

Compliance

A unique aspect of compliance with pediatric administration of analgesics is the use of patient controlled analgesia (PCA). Small children and infants may not have the cognitive ability or dexterity to successfully administer their own doses. As with adult patients, it is recommended that caregivers *not* administer boluses for the patient based on perceived need. This bypasses the safety of the PCA in that sedated patients can no longer add to their sedation by pressing the button for additional doses. Thus, PCA administration is not an option in small children. Determining when a PCA device can be used will vary based on the age, size, and cognitive ability of the child. Generally, when a patient is old enough to play video games, the patient is able to successfully use a PCA device.

Drug-specific information

The following safety pearls should be considered when administering analgesic and sedative agents:

Midazolam: Paradoxical reactions can occur (increased alertness); heparin and low serum protein can increase sedative effects.

Diazepam and lorazepam: These contain benzyl alcohol and/or propylene glycol that can cause toxicity in pediatric patients receiving continuous infusions. Neonates and small children are particularly at risk for toxicity.

Propofol: This is not recommended for routine sedation in pediatric patients due to the risk of the documented propofol-infusion syndrome (metabolic acidosis with cardiac failure); lipid emulsion increases risk of bacterial contamination, requiring tubing changes every 12 hours; must be avoided in soybean, egg glycerol, and disodium edetate allergies.

Barbiturates: Their narrow therapeutic index requires monitoring of levels; may actually increase sensitivity to pain.

Etomidate: This can be confused with dexmedetomidine. Although both are sedative agents, their effects are very different.

Chloral hydrate: This can cause a build-up of active and potentially toxic metabolites in neonates—avoid scheduled, chronic dosing. This is a poor choice for sedation due to its unpredictable onset and no available reversal agent.

Haloperidol: This can prolong QT interval and cause fatal arrhythmias—use caution in cardiac patients and with other medications that can prolong the QT interval. Patients receiving IV haloperidol should be monitored to detect any changes in heart rhythm.

Diphenhydramine: This is not recommended in patients younger than one year of age due to the dehydrating effects of its anticholinergic action; tolerance builds to sedative effects after a few days of use.

Morphine: Significant histamine release can cause hypotension—use caution in cardiac patients.

Meperidine: This can be metabolized to a toxic metabolite that can lead to seizures—avoid use; provides less pain relief and contributes to higher abuse potential compared to other available opiates.

Fentanyl: Chest wall rigidity can affect respiratory function and the ability to provide chest compressions in a code situation. Tolerance may build more rapidly than with longer-acting opiates such as morphine.

Methadone: It is difficult to convert to an equivalent dose from fentanyl when used in a sedation weaning regimen; long half-life may lead to accumulation and oversedation with frequent dosing.

Hydromorphone: This drug is seven times more potent than morphine, yet it is often inappropriately ordered using morphine doses due to similar sounding name. Giving hydromorphone at a typical morphine dose to an opiate naïve patient can result in serious respiratory depression.

Codeine: This can also be used for antitussive effects at lower oral doses—use caution to select appropriate dosing range for desired indication.

Hydrocodone: This is usually combined with acetaminophen—care must be taken not to cause an acetaminophen overdose if separate orders for acetaminophen are written for PRN fever or pain.

Oxycodone: Long-acting dosage forms can result in overdoses in children; be careful not to use a long-acting agent on a short-acting schedule (e.g., a twice-daily agent administered every 4 hours)

Ketamine: This is often used in acute asthma due to bronchodilation, but it can actually worsen respiratory secretions and airway responsiveness; uncomfortable emergence reactions can occur in children—concomitant use of a benzodiazepine is recommended while ketamine is being used and being discontinued.

Clonidine: Dose titration is required upon discontinuation due to rebound hypertension, yet it is difficult with limited dosage form availability for pediatric patients; patches must NEVER be cut to provide smaller doses.

Dexmedetomidine: This drug causes significant hypotension with loading doses and rebound hypertension with rapid discontinuation—avoid loading doses and wean off over several days in pediatric patients.

Aspirin: Avoid use in pediatric patients, *especially* in patients with viral infections due to the increased risk of Reye's Syndrome. Although Reye's Syndrome is a rare disorder that is not clearly caused by aspirin, the fatal increase in intracranial pressure definitely warrants careful consideration before use in the pediatric population (Orlowski 2002, Bhutta 2003)

Acetaminophen: Pay close attention to total daily acetaminophen dose when a patient has multiple orders of various formulations for various indications; include a max dose per day on order. Fatal liver failure can occur when patients receive acute or chronic overdoses of this common over-the-counter product.

Ketorolac: Duration of therapy must be limited to five days or less due to risk of GI bleeding.

Ibuprofen, naproxen: These can inhibit the antiplatelet activity of aspirin when given prior to aspirin. For maximum antiplatelet effect of aspirin, give 30 minutes before or 8 hours after ibuprofen or naproxen (Micromedex).

Nursing implications

Patients and families rely on healthcare providers—especially nurses—to protect them and keep them as comfortable as possible, as well as advocate for their needs. Accurate pain assessment is an essential component of a successful and safe pediatric pain management plan but is often difficult when caring for infants and young children. Therefore, pediatric nurses must excel at anticipating potentially painful interventions as well as supporting ongoing or long term comfort needs.

General pediatric pain principles

- ✓ Use age and developmentally appropriate pain tools to assess and document pain scores and to help guide pain management interventions (Potts & Mandleco 2007).

- ✓ Use nonpharmacological, age-appropriate interventions in combination with any pharmacological treatments to comfort a child who is experiencing pain (Potts & Mandleco 2007).

- ✓ If a procedure, intervention, or diagnosis is painful to an older child or adult, one must assume it is also painful—if not more painful—to young children and infants, even if they cannot verbally communicate their pain.

✓ Ask about previous experience with analgesic medications, including any side effects or adverse events.

✓ Recognize that one of a child's greatest fears is "getting a shot." If the pain management plan includes injections, or multiple IV sticks were needed to obtain an IV, a verbal child may be reluctant to admit to having any pain or needing pain medications.

✓ Consult with pharmacy experts for help with oral-to-IV conversions of opiates.

✓ With a few exceptions, medications administered using a patch are not recommended for pediatric patients. NEVER cut a patch in an attempt to administer a smaller dose. If a smaller dose than the commercially available sizes is needed, the safer way to administer a smaller dose is to occlude a portion of the patch with a clean dressing.

✓ Patient-controlled analgesia (PCA) is often an effective pain management strategy in older pediatric patients.

✓ Have the appropriate reversal agents available, including syringes and any equipment necessary for administration. Calculate the appropriate dose in advance to save time in the event that reversal is required.

Pain management safety considerations

Procedural pain management

✓ Involve the family or primary caregiver(s), whenever possible. Instruct them on ways they can assist to comfort their child during the procedure (Bowden & Greenberg 1998; Potts & Mandleco 2007). Tell them what they can expect to happen once the child has received the pain medication—such as whether the child is going to become sleepy or silly—so that they are not frightened and can be supportive.

✓ Tell children, using age-appropriate and developmentally focused language and preparation methods, what is going to happen, what they can expect, and what their role is during the procedure. A Child Life Specialist, if available, can be extremely helpful in assisting to prepare a child and his or her family for procedures.

✓ If the child must remain still during a painful procedure, consider adding a pediatric sedation agent.

✓ Recognize that when an analgesic and a sedative agent are used in combination, they provide a synergistic effect and the child may be at increased risk for adverse effects.

✓ Know the potential side effects of the medication being prescribed. Common side effects include (Bowden & Greenberg 1998):

- Respiratory depression

- Airway obstruction

- Oversedation

- Cardiac arrhythmias

- Hypotension

- Hypertension

✓ Have emergency equipment available.

Continuous or long-term pain management

✓ Patients on a continuous infusion who are undergoing a procedure may need additional bolus medication prior to the start of the procedure. Be prepared to increase the level of monitoring, if necessary.

✓ Administer bolus doses from pharmacy dispensed syringes, not from infusion bags or syringes (ISMP).

✓ PCAs should be used only in older school-age or adolescent patients. Provide patients and families with education about the goal of PCA pain management, how to use the PCA, and their role in the PCA pain management plan. PCA by proxy—such as medication administered because the nurse or a family member pushed the PCA—can result in unintended oversedation and should be discouraged. A continuous infusion and/or PRN dosing should be considered if the PCA method is ineffective.

✓ Monitor patients for signs of withdrawal or tolerance. This is difficult because these signs are often similar to signs of pain or agitation.

✓ Recognize the tolerance factor, and take it into consideration when weaning and/or increasing continuous infusions.

✓ Consult with pharmacy, the Child Life Specialist (if available), the child, the family, or the primary care providers and the primary care team to develop pain management plans for complex, chronic, or long-term pain challenges.

General pediatric sedation principles

✓ Ask about previous sedation experiences, including any side effects or adverse events.

✓ Consent is required for procedural sedation; continuous sedation is often part of emergency or life-threatening care interventions.

✓ Moderate sedation is used for interventions that may be painful and/or require the child to be perfectly still for the duration of the test or therapy.

✓ If a procedure or intervention could be painful, an analgesic must be administered along with the sedation medication (e.g., bone marrow aspiration, central line placement or bronchoscopy).

✓ Sometimes a child merely needs to be still. In these cases, sedation medications alone may be appropriate (e.g., MRI or PET scan).

✓ Persons caring for children during moderate sedation must have received competency-based training (Bowden & Greenberg 1998).

✓ At least one person must have the sole responsibility of monitoring and continuously assessing the patient throughout the procedure. If the person performing the procedure or intervention

Case study

Extra dosing

Ryan is a 3.5 kg baby who has just returned from the OR to the NICU following surgery for a gastrointestinal obstruction. He is ventilated, has a peripheral arterial line in his left hand, and is receiving intravenous fluids via a central line. While getting him settled in the NICU, Ryan's nurse notices that he is beginning to arouse from his anesthesia and alerts the neonatologist to Ryan's increasing pain score. The physician orders a fentanyl bolus 7 mcg slow IVP over two minutes (2 mcg/kg) as well as a continuous infusion using the available NICU standard concentration to run at 2 mcg/kg/hour.

Case study

The nurse administers the bolus dose, and Ryan appears to be more comfortable and his pain scores quickly decrease. The continuous infusion arrives, and using smart-pump infusion technology, the nurse begins the infusion. The unit is busy, so the nurse does not want to bother another nurse to double-check her infusion, and after all, the smart-pump technology should catch any errors made during the programming. The nurse continues to care for Ryan postoperatively, including assisting with a chest x-ray, drawing labs, and beginning new fluids via the central line, and updating Ryan's parents at the bedside. Soon it is change of shift, and Ryan's nurse gives a report to the oncoming night nurse. The nurses review Ryan's case, including his recent orders, but fail to double-check his continuous infusions. During evening rounds, the physician notices that Ryan's blood gases are worsening, his ventilator settings have been rapidly increasing, and his chest rise is severely decreased with poor air entry. The night physician asks how much fentanyl Ryan is receiving, and upon examining the infusion pump, notices that the pump is set to deliver the appropriate dose of 2 mcg/kg/hour; however, the standard concentration sent by the pharmacy is double the concentration that was originally ordered. Although the syringe is quickly discontinued, Ryan continues to require significant respiratory support throughout the shift. He is eventually restarted on the correct concentration and dose.

1. What critical safety steps were overlooked that could have prevented this error?

2. What processes do you have in place in your institution to prevent errors such as this from occurring?

3. Describe how you would approach Ryan's parents to explain this error.

requires assistance, a third person must be called so that the child is never left unattended or unobserved (Bowden & Greenberg 1998).

✓ Persons performing pediatric moderate sedation must be certified in either Pediatric Advanced Life Support (PALS) or Neonatal Resuscitation Program (NRP) (Bowden & Greenberg 1998).

✓ Emergency equipment must be available in any area where pediatric sedation is performed. Most institutional policies define required equipment. Universal requirements include (Bowden & Greenberg 1998):

  – Sedation documentation record

  – Continuous ECG and pulse oximetry monitoring

  – End-tidal CO_2/capnography monitoring

  – Blood pressure cuff and monitoring equipment

  – Supplemental oxygen, bag, and mask

  – Intubation and other airway maintenance equipment

  – Suction and suction equipment

  – Stethoscope

  – Pediatric emergency cart, including all emergency drugs and additional emergency equipment, if needed

✓ Assess the child's tolerance of the procedure using age-appropriate pain scales, vital signs, and any movements that indicate pain, anxiety, or discomfort.

Sedation safety considerations

Procedural sedation

✓ Involve the family or primary caregiver(s), whenever possible. Instruct them on their role during sedation induction and throughout any procedures (Bowden & Greenberg 1998; Potts & Mandleco 2007).

✓ Prior to the start of the sedation induction, tell them what they can expect to happen so that they are able to comfort the child and are not frightened or panicked when the sedation induction begins.

✓ Tell children, using age-appropriate and developmentally focused language and preparation methods, what is going to happen, what they can expect, and what their role is during the sedation procedure. A Child Life Specialist, if available, can be extremely helpful in assisting to prepare a child and his or her family for procedures.

✓ Document the last time the child had anything to eat or drink (Bowden & Greenberg 1998)

✓ Often, more than one medication is used for procedures requiring moderate sedation. Ensure correct medication, correct dose, correct route, and correct method of administration (e.g., slow IVP, rapid IVP, or infusion over time).

✓ Know the reversal agent and have it available.

✓ Record baseline vital signs and assessment findings prior to administering sedation medication (Bowden & Greenberg 1998).

✓ Perform continuous monitoring and routine documentation of assessment throughout the procedure, immediately following the procedure, and during the recovery phase (per institutional policy).

✓ Warn parents that sometimes children may be crying or irritable when waking up from sedation, and that this is often expected and will diminish as the medication effects continue to wear off.

✓ Recognize the potential complications of sedation and be prepared to address them immediately, if needed (Bowden & Greenberg 1998).

Continuous sedation

Continuous sedation mediations are most often used in conjunction with analgesic agent to support comfort during prolonged sedation.

✓ Continuously support and assess respiratory status

✓ Continuously monitor ECG, oxygen saturations, blood pressure, and capnography

✓ Depth of sedation should be regularly monitored and documented according to institutional policy and available technologies

✓ Administer bolus doses from pharmacy dispensed syringes, not from infusion bags or syringes (ISMP)

Case study

Oversedation

An 18-month-old presented in the ED with a skull fracture following an accidental fall from a neighbor's deck. A CT scan was ordered as part of her evaluation. The child was active, crying, and difficult to console in the ED. Chloral hydrate (50 mg/kg/dose) was ordered to help keep her calm and to keep her from moving during the CT scan. The toddler weighed 11 kg and was given 550 mg PO 30 minutes prior to the procedure. Upon arriving in the CT department, she was still active and crying and unwilling to let go of her mother to be laid in the scanner. An additional 50 mg/kg/dose (550 mg) was given PO. After approximately 20 minutes, she began to grow sleepy. She was placed on the CT table, a pulse oximeter was placed on her finger, and she was slowly moved into the scanner for the start of the test. Soon after the pulse oximeter was attached, the reading became erratic, bouncing from an SaO_2 of 96% to what the nurse and tech defined as artifact, and then reading the child's SaO_2 and blinking off again. The nurse assumed this was occurring because the child was occasionally moving, and therefore an accurate, consistent reading could not be obtained. The tech assured the nurse the test was almost complete and that she could fix the probe as soon as the scan ended. Upon completion of the test, the child was removed from the scanner. She was found to be pale and limp with no respiratory effort. A pediatric code was called, and following a lengthy resuscitation effort, the child was pronounced dead less than one hour after the start of the CT scan.

1. What could have been done to prevent this fatal pediatric sedation error?

2. What processes and policies do you have in place in your institution to help keep children safe during procedural sedation?

Appreciation for unique aspects of treating pediatric pain and sedation, understanding appropriate drug selection, and careful attention to monitoring are essential elements for the safe use of analgesics and sedatives in pediatric patients.

Bibliography

References

Alton, M., K. Frush, D. Brandon, and J. Mericle. (2006). "Development and implementation of a pediatric patient safety program." *Advances in Neonatal Care* 6(3): 104–111.

Alemzadeh, R., and D. Wyatt. (2004). "Diabetes mellitus" in *Nelson's Textbook of Pediatrics* 4th Edition. Philadelphia: W.B. Saunders.

American Academy of Pediatrics, Committee on Drugs and Committee on Hospital Care. (2003). "Prevention of medication errors in the pediatric inpatient setting." *Pediatrics* 112(2): 431–436.

American Academy of Pediatrics, Committee on Psychosocial Aspects of Child and Family Health. (2001). "The assessment and management of acute pain in infants, children, and adolescents." *Pediatrics* 108: 793–7.

American Academy of Pediatrics, Committee on Nutrition. (1976). "Commentary on breast-feeding and infant formulas, including proposed standards for formulas." *Pediatrics* 57: 278–285.

American Society of Health-System Pharmacists (ASHP). (2004.) *Competency Assessment Tools for Health-system Pharmacies*, third edition. Bethesda, MD: ASHP.

American Society of Health-System Pharmacists (ASHP). (2007). "Professional practice recommendations for safe use of insulin in hospitals: A joint project of the American Society of Health-System Pharmacists and the Hospital and Health-System Association of Pennsylvania." Available at *www.ashp.org/s_ashp/docs/files/Safe_Use_of_Insulin.pdf*.

American Society for Parenteral and Enteral Nutrition (ASPEN). (1998). "Safe practices for parenteral nutrition formulations." *Journal of Parenteral and Enteral Nutrition* March/April 1998: 72–78.

Anand, KJ. "Consensus statement for the prevention and management of pain in the newborn." *Archives of Pediatric Adolescent Medicine* 155(2): 173–180.

Bhatt-Mehta, V., and D. Rosen. (1998). "Sedation in children: Current concepts." *Pharmacotherapy* 18(4): 790–807.

Bhutta, A., H. Van Savell, and S. Schexnayder. (2003). "Reye's syndrome: Down but not out." *Southern Medical Journal* 96(1): 43–5.

Brandom, B., and G. Fine. (2002). "Neuromuscular blocking agents in paediatric anaesthesia." *Anesthesiology Clinics of North America* 20(1):45–58.

Bowden, V., and C. Smith-Greenberg (1998). *Pediatric Nursing Procedures* (2nd ed). Philadelphia: Lippincott Williams & Wilkins.

Centers for Disease Control and Prevention (CDC). (2002). "Fact sheet: Hand hygiene guidelines fact sheet." Available at *www.cdc.gov/od/oc/media/pressrel/fs021025.htm.*

Chambliss, C., and K. Anand. (1997). "Pain management in the pediatric intensive care unit." *Current Opinion in Pediatrics* 9: 246–53.

DeWitt, D., and I. Hirsch. (2003). "Outpatient insulin therapy in type 1 and type 2 diabetes mellitus." *The Journal of the American Medical Association* 289(17): 2254–2264.

Dickerson, R, and G. Melnik. (1998). "Osmolality of oral drug solutions and suspensions." *American Journal of Hospital Pharmacy* 45(4): 832–4.

Doniger, S., and G. Sharieff. (2006). "Pediatric dysrhythmias." *Pediatric Clinics of North America* 53: 85–105.

Elgart, H. (2004). "Assessment of fluids and electrolytes." *AACN Clinical Issues* 15(4): 607–621.

Erstad, B. "Osmolality and osmolarity: Narrowing the terminology gap." *Pharmacotherapy* 23(9): 1085–1086.

Federal Drug Administration. (2004). Federal Food, Drug, and Cosmetic Act. Available at *www.fda.gov.*

Fisher, D. (1999). "Neuromuscular blocking agents." *British Journal of Anaesthesia* 83: 58–64.

Fortescue, E., R. Kaushal, C. Landrigan, et al. (2003). "Prioritizing strategies for preventing medication errors and adverse drug events in pediatric patients." *Pediatrics* 111(4): 722–279.

Gaylor, A., and M. Condren. (2004). "Type 2 diabetes mellitus in the pediatric population." *Pharmacotherapy* 24(7): 871–878.

Harder, A. (2002). "The developmental stages of Erik Erikson." Available at *www.support4change.com/ stages/cycles/Erikson.html.*

Harrison, A., R. Lugo, W. Lee, E. Appachi, et al. (2002). "The use of haloperidol in agitated critically ill children." *Clinical Pediatrics* 41(1): 51–4.

Hazinski, M. (1991). *Nursing Care of the Critically Ill Child* (2nd ed.) St. Louis: Mosby.

Hirsch, I. (2005). "Insulin analogues." *New England Journal of Medicine* 352: 174–183.

Hockenberry, M., and D. Wilson. (2007). *Wong's Nursing Care of Infants & Children,* 8th edition. St. Louis: Mosby.

Hughes, R., and E. Edgerton (2005). "First, do no harm: Reducing pediatric medication errors: Children are especially at risk for medication errors." *American Journal of Nursing* 105(5): 79–84.

Institute for Healthcare Improvement (IHI). (2007). "Reduce adverse drug events involving anticoagulants." Available from *www.ihi.org.*

Institute for Healthcare Improvement (IHI). (2007). "Reduce adverse drug events involving chemotherapy." Available from *www.ihi.org.*

Institute for Healthcare Improvement (IHI). (2007). "Reduce adverse drug events involving electrolytes." Available at *www.ihi.org.*

Institute for Healthcare Improvement (IHI). (2007). "Reduce adverse drug events involving insulin." Available at *www.ihi.org.*

Institute for Safe Medication Practices. *www.ismp.org.*

Institute for Safe Medication Practices. (2007). "Historical timeline." Available at *www.ismp.org*.

Institute for Safe Medication Practices. (2007). "Lack of standard dosing methods contributes to IV errors." *Medication Safety Alert* August 23. Available at *www.ismp.org*.

Institute for Safe Medication Practices. (2007). "List of high-alert medications." Available at *www.ismp.org*.

Institute for Safe Medication Practices. (2006). September 2006. "Infant heparin flush overdose." Available at *www.ismp.org*.

Institute for Safe Medication Practices. (2005). "Fatal misadministration of IV vincristine." *Medication Safety Alert* December 1. Available at *www.ismp.org*.

Institute for Safe Medication Practices. (2005). "Paralyzed by mistakes: Preventing errors with neuromuscular blocking agents." *Medication Safety Alert* September 22. Available at *www.ismp.org*.

Institute for Safe Medication Practices. (2004.) "Improvised drug delivery: A cause for concern." *Medication Safety Alert* April. Available at *www.ismp.org*.

Institute for Safe Medication Practices. (2003). "The virtues of independent double checks—they really are worth your time!" *Medication Safety Alert* March. Available at *www.ismp.org*.

Institute for Safe Medication Practices. (2000). "Hospital survey shows much more needs to be done to protect pediatric patients from medication errors." (2000). *Medication Safety Alert* April 19. Available at *www.ismp.org*.

Institute for Safe Medication Practices. (1997). "Which IV calcuim: Chloride or gluconate?" *Medication Safety Alert* May 7. Available at *www.ismp.org*.

Jew, R. (1997). "A modified version of osmolality of commonly used medications and formulas in the neonatal intensive care unit." *Nutrition in Clinical Practice* 12:158.

Kaushal, R, D. Bates, C. Landrigan, K. McKenna, et al. (2001). "Medication errors and adverse drug events in pediatric inpatients." *The Journal of the American Medical Association* 285(16): 2114–2120.

Kaushal, R., K. Barker, D. Bates. (2001). "How can information technology improve patient safety and reduce medication errors in children's health care?" *Archives of Pediatric Adolescent Medicine* 155: 1002–1007.

Kim, G., A. Chen, R. Arceci, S. Mitchell, et al. (2006). "Error reduction in pediatric chemotherapy." *Archives of Pediatric Adolescent Medicine* 160: 495–498.

Kline, N., et al. (2004). *Essentials of Pediatric Oncology Nursing: A Core Curriculum* (2nd ed.). Glenview, IL: Association of Pediatric Oncology Nurses.

Kraft, M., I. Btaiche, and G. Sacks. (2005). "Review of the refeeding syndrome." *Nutrition in Clinical Practice* 20(6): 625–633.

Kozer, E, M. Berkovitch, and G. Koren. (2006). "Medication errors in children." *Pediatric Clinics of North America* 53: 1155–1168.

Larsen et al. (2005). "Standard drug concentrations and smart-pump technology reduce continuous-medication-infusion errors in pediatric patients." *Pediatrics* 116: e21–e25.

Lefrack, L. et al. (2006). "Sucrose analgesia: Identifying potentially better practices." *Pediatrics* 118, Supplement 2066: S197–S202.

Levine, S. et al. (2001). "Guidelines for preventing medication errors in pediatrics." *The Journal of Pediatric Pharmacology and Therapeutics* 6: 426–442.

Lesar, T.S. (1998). "Errors in the use of medication dosage equations." *Archives of Pediatric Adolescent Medicine* 152(4): 340–344.

Lexi-Comp. (2006). Electronic Database 2006. Available at *www.lexi.com*.

Liem, R., M. Higman, A. Chen, and R. Arceci. (2003). "Misinterpretation of a calvert-derived formula leading to carboplatin overdose in two children." *Journal of Pediatric Hematology Oncology* 25(10): 818–821.

McKenry, L., E. Tessier, and M. Hogan. (2005). *Pharmacology in Nursing* (22nd edition). St. Louis: Mosby.

McPhillips, H., C. Stille, D. Smith, J. Hecht, et al. (2005) "Potential medication dosing errors in outpatient pediatrics." *Journal of Pediatrics* 147: 761–7.

Miller-Hoover, S. (2003). "Pediatric and neonatal cardiovascular pharmacology." *Pediatric Nursing* 29(2): 105–115.

Miller, M., K. Robinson, L. Lubomski, M. Rinke, and P. Pronovost (2007). "Medication errors in paediatric care: A systematic review of epidemiology and an evaluation of evidence supporting reduction strategy recommendations." *Quality and Safety in Health Care* 16: 116–126.

Mitchell, A. (2001). "Challenges in pediatric pharmacotherapy: Minimizing medication errors." *Medscape Pharmacists* 2(1). Available at *www.medscape.com/viewarticle/421220*.

Monagle, P., A. Chan, P. Massicotte, E. Chalmers, and A. Michelson. (2004). "Antithrombotic therapy in children: The seventh ACCP conference on antithrombotic and thrombolytic therapy." *Chest* 126(3): 645–687.

Monagle, P. (2004). "Anticoagulation in the young." *Heart* 90: 808–812.

Murphy, J. (2001). *Clinical Pharmacokinetics* Second Edition. Bethesda, MD: ASHP.

National Diabetes Education Program. (2004). "An update on type 2 diabetes in youth from the national diabetes education program." *Pediatrics* 114: 259–263.

Odland, H., E. Thaulow. (2006). "Heart failure therapy in children." *Expert Review of Cardiovascular Therapy* 4(1): 33–40.

Ohno, T. (1988). *The Toyota Production System: Beyond Large-Scale Production.* Cambridge, MA: Productivity Press.

Orlowski, J., U. Hanhan, and M. Fiallos (2002). "Is aspirin a cause of Reye's syndrome? A case against." *Drug Safety* 25(4): 225–31.

Payne, C, C. Smith, L. Newkirk, R. Hicks. (2007). "Pediatric medication errors in the postanesthesia care unit: Analysis of MEDMARX data." *AORN Journal* 85(4): 731–740.

Potts, N., and B. Mandleco (2007). *Pediatric Nursing: Caring for Children and Their Families* (2nd ed) Clifton Park, NY: Thomson Delmar Learning.

Rinke, M., A. Shore, L. Morlock, R. Hicks, and M. Miller. (2007). "Characteristics of pediatric chemotherapy medication errors in a national error reporting database." *Cancer* 110(1): 186–195.

Roberts, K. (2001). "Fluid and electrolytes: Parenteral fluid therapy." *Pediatrics in Review* 22: 380–387.

Robertson, J., and N. Shilkofski. (2005). *Harriet Lane Handbook,* 17th Edition. St. Louis: Mosby.

Rodriguez, E., and R. Jordan. (2002). "Contemporary trends in pediatric sedation and analgesia." *Emergency Medicine Clinics of North America* 20(1): 199–222.

Ronghe, M., C. Halsey, and N. Goulden N. (2003). "Anticoagulation therapy in children." *Pediatric Drugs* 5(12): 803–820.

Rowland, J. (2005). "Foreward: Looking beyond cure: Pediatric cancer as a model." *Journal of Pediatric Psychology* 30(1): 1–3.

Schneppenheim, R., and J. Greiner. (2006). "Thrombosis in infants and children." *Hematology* 2006: 86–96.

Scott, G. and Elmer, G. (2002). "Update on natural product-drug interactions." *American Journal of Health-System Pharmacy* 59(4): 339–347.

Simbre, V., S. Duffy, G. Dadlani, T. Miller, and S. Lipshultz. (2005). "Cardiotoxicity of cancer chemotherapy: Implications for children." *Paediatric Drugs* 7(3): 187–202.

Slota, M. (2006). *Core Curriculum for Pediatric Critical Care Nursing* (2nd ed.). Philadelphia: Saunders.

Smetzer, J. (1998). "Lessons from Colorado: Beyond blaming individuals." *Nursing* June; 29(6): 49–51.

Taketomo, C., et al. (2005). *Pediatric Dosage Handbook: Including Neonatal Dosing, Drug Administration, & Extemporaneous Preparations,* 13th edition. Hudson, OH: Lexi-Comp.

Tang, J., and S. Gibson. (2005). "A psychophysical evaluation of the relationship between trait anxiety, pain perception, and induced state anxiety." *The Journal of Pain* 6(9): 612–9.

Taylor, J., L. Winter, L. Geyer, and D. Hawkins. (2006). "Oral outpatient chemotherapy medication errors in children with acute lymphoblastic leukemia." *Cancer* 107(6): 1400–1406.

The Joint Commission. (2007). "2008 National Patient Safety Goals: Facts about the 2008 National Patient Safety Goals." Available at *www.jointcommission.org.*

The Joint Commission. (2006). "2007 National Patient Safety Goals: Facts about the 2007 National Patient Safety Goals." Available at *www.jointcommission.org.*

The Joint Commission. (2007) "Facts about the official do not use list". Available at *www.jointcommission.org.*

The Josie King Foundation. Available at *www.josieking.org.*

Thomas, D. (2005). "Lessons learned: Basic evidence-based advice for preventing medication errors in children." *Journal of Emergency Nursing* 31(5): 490–493.

Thomson Healthcare. (2007). *Micromedex® Healthcare Series.* Available from *www.micromedex.com.*

Tobias, J. (1999). "Sedation and analgesia in paediatric intensive care units." *Paediatric Drugs* 1(2): 109–126.

Topps, C., et al. (2005). "Perceptions of pediatric nurses toward bar-code point-of-care medication administration." *Nursing Administration Quarterly* 29(1): 102–107.

Wang, J, N. Herzog, R. Kaushal, C. Park, et al. (2007). "Prevention of pediatric medication errors by hospital pharmacists and the potential benefit of computerized physician order entry." *Pediatrics* 119(1): e77–e85.

WHO Collaborating Centre for Patient Safety Solutions. (2007). "Control of concentrated electrolyte solutions." *Patient Safety Solutions* 1(5).

Williams, R., and D. Dunger. (2003). "Insulin treatment in children and adolescents." *Acta* Paediatr 93(4): 440–446.

Yaffe, S, & J. Aranda. (2005). *Neonatal and Pediatric Pharmacology: Therapeutic Principles in Practice,* Third Edition. Philadelphia: Lippincott Williams & Wilkins.

Young, T., and B. Mangum. (2007). *NeoFax 2007.* Thomson Healthcare. Available at *http://neofax.com/.*

Nursing education instructional guide

Pediatric High-Alert Medications: Evidence-Based Safe Practices for Nursing

Target audience

Chief Nursing Officers

Directors of Nursing

Nurse Managers

Staff educators

Staff nurses

Statement of need

According to the Institute for Healthcare Improvement (IHI), adverse drug events occur in 6% to 10% of all hospitalized patients, and each year thousands of patients die from drug-related injuries. High-alert medications are drugs that have a greater risk of causing significant patient harm when they are used in error and nurses need specific training on these medications. Children react differently to drugs than adults, so there is a need for pediatric specific information as children are more likely to be harmed by adverse drug events than adults. (This activity is intended for individual use only.)

Educational objectives

Upon completion of this activity, participants should be able to:

- Identify the key differences in providing pharmaceutical care to pediatric patients

- Recognize the importance of a systems approach to medication safety in pediatric patients

- Explain the special considerations necessary when formulating adult dosage forms for pediatric administration

- Identify the "six Rights" of safe pediatric high-alert medication administration

- Describe the role that The Joint Commission's National Patient Safety Goals play in pediatric high-alert medication safety initiatives

- Identify the role that error reporting plays in improving pediatric high-alert medication safety

- Describe the role technology plays in pediatric high-alert medication safety

- Identify at least two recent technological advances found to be effective in preventing pediatric medication errors

- Identify at least two pharmacy processes that can improve pediatric high-alert medication safety

- Recognize the safety implications of using the correct syringe type for oral and intravenous medications

- Illustrate child-friendly and developmentally friendly techniques that are useful when administering medications to children ranging in age from infancy through adolescence

- Recognize why anticoagulant medications are considered pediatric high-alert medications

- Describe the anticoagulant medications most commonly used in pediatric patients

- Identify at least three ways to prevent errors when administering anticoagulant medications to pediatric patients

- Recognize why chemotherapeutic agents are considered pediatric high-alert medications

- Describe the chemotherapeutic agents most commonly used in pediatric patients

- Identify at least three ways to prevent errors when administering chemotherapeutic agents to pediatric patients

- Recognize why concentrated electrolytes are considered pediatric high-alert medications

- Describe the concentrated electrolytes most commonly used in pediatric patients

- Identify at least three ways to prevent errors when administering concentrated electrolytes to pediatric patients

- Recognize why cardiovascular medications are considered pediatric high-alert medications

- Describe the cardiovascular medications most commonly used in pediatric patients

- Identify at least three ways to prevent errors when administering cardiovascular medications to pediatric patients

- Recognize why insulin and concentrated dextrose solution are considered pediatric high-alert medications

- Describe the insulin and concentrated dextrose solution most commonly used in pediatric patients

- Identify at least three ways to prevent errors when administering insulin and concentrated dextrose solution to pediatric patients

- Recognize why neuromuscular blockers (NMB) are considered a pediatric high-alert medication

- Describe the NMBs most commonly used in pediatric patients

- Identify at least three ways to prevent errors when administering NMBs to pediatric patients

- Recognize why some medications used to treat pediatric pain and provide sedation are considered pediatric high-alert medications

- Describe the classes of medication used for pain and sedation treatment in pediatric patients

- Identify at least three ways to prevent errors when administering pain medications to pediatric patients

- List at least five common safety components of any pediatric sedation program

Faculty

Jill Duncan, RN, MS, MPH, is the clinical nurse specialist for the neonatal intensive care unit (NICU) at Inova Fairfax Hospital for Children in Falls Church, VA. She has more than 14 years of pediatric-related experience in a variety of acute care settings, including the National Institutes of Health (NIH).

She received her master's of science and master's of public health degrees with a focus in maternal and child health from the University of Illinois at Chicago in 2000 and received her bachelor of science in nursing from Georgetown University in Washington, DC, in 1993. Her professional memberships include the National Association of Neonatal Nurses and The Academy of Neonatal Nursing. She was featured in an Academy of Neonatal Nursing member spotlight in 2007. The same publication also highlighted the collaborative work she has done on the development of a virtual NICU critical decision simulation education program for nurses. She is also an active volunteer with the March of Dimes, National Capital Area Chapter.

Jason Corcoran, PharmD, BCPS, is the clinical pharmacy specialist for Inova Fairfax Hospital for Children in Falls Church, VA. He has more than 10 years of pharmacy work experience, including the past five years in practice as a pediatric pharmacist.

In his current role at Inova Fairfax, he provides clinical pharmacy oversight for 186 pediatric beds comprising the pediatric intensive care, neonatal intensive care, pediatric medical-surgical, pediatric hematology-oncology, pediatric emergency, and adolescent units. Corcoran received his doctor of pharmacy degree from Virginia Commonwealth University based in Richmond in 2001. He is a member of pharmaceutical organizations including the American Society of Health Systems Pharmacists and the American College of Clinical Pharmacy. As a member of the Pediatric Pharmacy Advocacy Group for the past five years he has twice been invited to speak at its national meetings. In 2005, he achieved board certification in pharmacotherapy, a qualification that recognizes additional knowledge, experience, and skills in a defined area of pharmacy practice.

Accreditation/Designation statement

HCPro, Inc. is accredited as a provider of continuing nursing education by the American Nurses Credentialing Center Commission on Accreditation.

This educational activity for three nursing contact hours is provided by HCPro, Inc.

Disclosure statements

HCPro, Inc., has a conflict of interest policy that requires course faculty to disclose any real or apparent commercial financial affiliations related to the content of their presentations/materials. It is not assumed that these financial interests or affiliations will have an adverse impact on faculty presentations; they are simply noted here to fully inform the participants.

Jill Duncan and Jason Corcoran have declared that they have no commercial/financial vested interest in this activity.

Instructions

In order to be eligible to receive your nursing contact hours for this activity, you are required to do the following:

1. Read the book, **Pediatric High-Alert Medications: Evidence-Based Safe Practices for Nursing**

2. Complete the exam

3. Complete the evaluation

4. Provide your contact information on the exam and evaluation

5. Submit exam and evaluation to HCPro, Inc.

Please provide all of the information requested above and mail or fax your completed exam, program evaluation, and contact information to

Kerry Betsold
Continuing Education Manager
HCPro, Inc.
200 Hoods Lane
P.O. Box 1168
Marblehead, MA 01945
Fax: 781/639-0179

NOTE:

This book and associated exam are intended for individual use only. If you would like to provide this continuing education exam to other members of your nursing staff, please contact our customer service department at 877/727-1728 to place your order. The exam fee schedule is as follows:

Number of exams	Fee
1	$0
2-25	$15 per person
26-50	$12 per person
51-100	$8 per person
101+	$5 per person

Continuing education exam

Name: _____

Title: _____

Facility Name: _____

Address: _____

Address: _____

City: _____ State: _____ ZIP: _____

Phone number: _____ Fax number: _____

E-mail: _____

Nursing license number: _____

(ANCC requires a unique identifier for each learner.)

Date completed: _____

1. The key physiologic difference between pediatric and adult patients includes all of the following, except:

    a. Pediatric patients have increased body mass and body surface area (BSA) per kilogram (kg) than adults

    b. The percentage of body water in pediatric patients decreases as age increases

    c. Glomerular filtration increases rapidly during the first two weeks of life, with continued improvement to adult values by six to 12 months of age

    d. Organs such as the brain and liver are proportionally smaller in pediatric patients

2. Which of the following is a reason that children are at a greater risk for drug-related problems?

a. Pediatric medications have better standardization and information on stability compared to adult medications

b. Small doses that require further dilution, calculations, or partial dosage forms have a greater likelihood of resulting in overdoses or ineffective doses

c. Children have fewer interruptions in dosing schedules

d. Children often do not receive enough fluid volume because doses are small, putting them at risk for hypovolemia

3. Not all medications come in a form that is suitable for pediatric patients. What is the ideal oral dosage form for pediatric patients?

a. Chewable, because you can fool a child into thinking it is candy

b. Capsules, because all types of capsules can be sprinkled in food and easily disguised

c. Liquid, because many children find it difficult, or simply refuse, to swallow solid medication

d. Extended-release tablets, because even if you crush them, they still retain their extended-release potency in children

4. The sixth "Right" of safe medication administration in pediatrics is:

a. The RIGHT patient

b. The RIGHT medication

c. The RIGHT route

d. The RIGHT age-appropriate approach, explanation, and administration techniques

5. A pediatric high-alert medication is one that is frequently prescribed, frequently given in error, and:

    a. Frequently tastes bad

    b. Is difficult to obtain

    c. Has a high risk of causing harm when used incorrectly

    d. Is not reimbursed by most insurance plans

6. Why do pediatric nurses need to know about The Joint Commission National Patient Safety Goals?

    a. Nurses are sued more frequently than doctors or pharmacists in legal cases related to medication errors

    b. The nurse is often the final step, or layer, in safe medication administration practices

    c. The National Patient Safety Goals are the best place to learn more about the differences between pediatric and adult medication administration

    d. Nurses do not need to be familiar with the National Patient Safety Goals because they relate only to prescribers and hospital administration

7. It is essential to report medication errors or adverse drug events because:

    a. We are better able to learn from our mistakes, improve our processes, and prevent errors from happening in the future

    b. By reporting errors to risk management, we do not have to tell the family

    c. Human resources needs to keep track of who makes mistakes and who doesn't

    d. Errors should be kept quiet; nothing good comes from reporting them

8. Technology works to improve pediatric high-alert medication safety by:

a. Providing a foolproof final check for all medication orders

b. Providing a sort of checks-and-balances system to guide users to make the correct choices and issuing alerts before an error is made

c. Decreasing the number of people that need to be involved in the medication processes

d. Serving as the double-check in most processes so that nurses do not have to bother a colleague to double-check medications prior to administration

9. Which of the following technologies evolved to help improve patient safety during the administration of standardized concentrated drips?

a. Bar-coding technology

b. CPOE technology

c. Preprinted order sheets

d. Smart-pump technology

10. Pharmacy unit dosing means:

a. The pharmacist writes all medication orders for pediatric patients

b. A pharmacist trained in pediatrics staffs the pharmacy

c. All orders are double-checked by a pediatric pharmacist

d. A pharmacist trained in pediatrics is responsible for preparing and dispensing the medication in a ready to administer formulation

11. Oral syringes improve pediatric medication safety by:

a. Eliminating the chance that oral medications could accidentally be connected to and administered into an IV site

b. Replacing IV syringes and therefore decreasing the cost of medication administration for pediatric patients

c. Offering a reusable alternative for pediatric medication administration

d. Decreasing the chance that the incorrect volume of medication will be administered

12. Applying age-appropriate and developmentally appropriate techniques to medication administration practices improves pediatric medication safety because:

   a. It is a requirement of The Joint Commission National Patient Safety Goals

   b. It supports the child's stage of development and the family's role in medication administration and compliance

   c. It helps to trick the child into thinking he or she is safe during medication administration times

   d. It means the nurse is the expert and therefore should always be the one to administer the child's medications

13. All of the following are reasons why anticoagulants are considered high-risk medications for pediatrics, but which reason is most critical?

   a. Look-alike, sound-alike names and packaging

   b. Need for multifaceted calculations

   c. Need for complex titrating regimens

   d. Narrow therapeutic index and potential to cause significant bleeding

14. Which of the following can be used as an oral anticoagulant?

   a. heparin

   b. enoxaparin

   c. warfarin

   d. lepirudin

15. Which of he following is an example of the correct way to order or document heparin?

   a. 1 unit/mL

   b. 1.0 unit/mL

   c. 1 u/mL

   d. 1.0 u/mL

16. Some of the documented problems that have prompted chemotherapeutic agents to now be considered pediatric high-alert medications include all of the following, EXCEPT:

    a. Unintentional overdose

    b. Inadvertent administration due to look-alike packaging or sound-alike medications

    c. Too much heparin added to chemotherapy solution

    d. Incorrect route during the administration

17. One of the problems that is NOT related to chemotherapeutic agents being considered pediatric high-alert medications is:

    a. Calculations required for proper dosing

    b. High potency

    c. Narrow therapeutic index

    d. Respiratory depression

18. "Stop the line" means:

    a. Discharge the patient immediately

    b. Discontinue the IV line immediately

    c. Stop the action or activity for safety reasons and review the process with everyone involved

    d. Stop the chemotherapy infusion

19. Electrolytes are often among the most lethal medications that are administered in a hospital setting, but the risk is overlooked partly because they are often not considered medications. Which one is NOT a common cause of errors with electrolytes?

    a. Patient preference

    b. Look-alike packaging

    c. Erroneous dispensing

    D. Infusion mistakes

20. A dose of 3% sodium chloride is ordered for a patient that is severely hyponatremic. What route(s) are considered safe for concentrated sodium administration?

a. Orally

b. IM

c. Peripherally

d. In a central line only

21. When administering concentrated electrolytes, you should:

a. Place the patient on continuous ECG and pulse oximetry monitors

b. Place the patient on continuous temperature monitoring

c. Situate the patient in the bed closest to the nurses' station

d. Tell the child's parents they cannot leave because they need to help monitor their child closely

22. Cardiovascular drugs are considered to be high-alert medications because they may cause cardiovascular parameters to be _____ than a normal range.

a. Higher

b. Lower

c. Higher or lower

d. About the same

23. Apnea associated with the administration of prostaglandin (PGE[1]) most often occurs:

a. After 24 hours

b. Within the first hour

c. After long-term use (>7 days)

d. Apnea is not associated with prostaglandin administration

24. Continuous medication infusion safety includes all of the following except:

a. Programming continuous infusion pumps and asking a coworker to double-check the rate after at least 1 hour has infused.

b. Ensuring that all infusion lines are clearly marked, including at connection ports closest to the patient

c. Avoiding infusing intermittent, IV-push, or piggyback medications through lines containing continuous infusion medications, as this could result in unintended surges or boluses

d. Labeling all continuous infusion bags or syringes clearly

25. Insulin is a high-alert medication for all of the following reasons except:

a. Look-alike packaging

b. Standardization of dosing

c. Different concentrations

d. Sound-alike names

26. Which of the following solutions is not safe to administer via a peripheral IV line?

a. D10W

b. D12W

c. D7.5W

d. D15W

27. When mixing regular insulin with other preparations, you should draw regular insulin into the syringe:

a. First

b. In between any additional insulin products

c. Last

d. Regular insulin should never be given SQ

28. NMBs are high-alert medications because they cause:

  a. Paralysis of the skeletal muscles, including the diaphragm

  b. Sedation

  c. Pain relief

  d. Patients to feel less anxiety

29. The physician wrote an order to extubate the child you are caring for but did not indicate any changes in the patient's medications. The patient is being treated with a continuous fentanyl, midozolam, and vecuronium drip. You should:

  a. Extubate the patient, as the order states

  b. Notify the physician immediately that the patient is still on a vecuronium drip and needs to have the medication discontinued prior to extubation

  c. Have a bag and mask ready just in case the patient needs oxygen following immediate extubation

  d. Have Narcan available in the event that a reversal agent is required

30. When treating a child with neuromuscular blocking (NMB) agents, it is essential to administer all of the following except:

  a. An analgesic, typically an opioid analgesic

  b. Nasal drops

  c. Eye lubrication

  d. An anti-anxiety medication, typically a benzodiazepem

31. Opiates are one of the ____ medications to cause patient harm.

  a. Most common

  b. Least common

  c. Most prescribed

  d. Least prescribed

32. Which of the following drugs is an opioid analgesic most commonly used in pediatric patients.

    a. midazolam

    b. ketorolac

    c. morphine

    d. chloral hydrate

33. Identify the most common side effects associated with opioid analgesic medications:

    a. Bradycardia and hypoglycemia

    b. Respiratory depression and apnea

    c. Hyperthermia and seizure

    d. Hypertension and bradycardia

34. While monitoring a child undergoing moderate sedation for a procedure in the ED, the physician asks for a piece of equipment located in another room. The correct response is:

    a. "I'll be right back. Please watch the monitor for me and document the vital signs."

    b. "I cannot leave the patient, but I will call someone else to assist."

    c. "I can step out just as soon as some of the medication wears off, and then we can begin again."

    d. "I will be right back. I just need to get the reversal agent to wake up the patient first."

Continuing education evaluation

Name: _____

Title: _____

Facility Name: _____

Address: _____

Address: _____

City: _____ State: _____ ZIP: _____

Phone number: _____ Fax number: _____

E-mail: _____

Nursing license number: _____

(ANCC requires a unique identifier for each learner.)

Date Completed: _____

1. This activity met the learning objectives stated:

Strongly Agree   Agree   Disagree   Strongly Disagree

2. Objectives were related to the overall purpose/goal of the activity:

Strongly Agree   Agree   Disagree   Strongly Disagree

3. This activity was related to my continuing education needs:

Strongly Agree   Agree   Disagree   Strongly Disagree

4. The exam for the activity was an accurate test of the knowledge gained:

Strongly Agree   Agree   Disagree   Strongly Disagree

5. The activity avoided commercial bias or influence:

       Strongly Agree   Agree   Disagree   Strongly Disagree

6. This activity met my expectations:

       Strongly Agree   Agree   Disagree   Strongly Disagree

7. Will this activity enhance your professional practice?

       Yes   No

8. The format was an appropriate method for delivery of the content for this activity:

       Strongly Agree   Agree   Disagree   Strongly Disagree

9. If you have any comments on this activity please note them here:

10. How much time did it take for you to complete this activity?

Thank you for completing this evaluation of our continuing education activity!

Return completed form to:

HCPro, Inc. · Attn: Kerry Betsold · 200 Hoods Lane, Marblehead, MA 01945
· Tel 877/727-1728
· Fax 781/639-2982